The Colostrum Miracle

Disclaimer: This information is presented by independent medical experts whose sources of information include studies from the world's medical and scientific literature, patient records, and other clinical and anecdotal reports. The material in this book is for informational purposes only and is not intended for the diagnosis or treatment of disease. Please visit a medical health professional for specific diagnosis of any ailments mentioned or discussed in this material.

Cover design by Bonnie Lambert
Book design by Debbie Wells

ISBN 1-893910-36-9
First printing
PRINTED IN CANADA
Published by Freedom Press
1801 Chart Trail
Topanga, CA 90290
Bulk Orders Available: (800) 959-9797
E-mail: info@freedompressonline.com

Contents

Foreword

It was my good fortune to serve 12 years in the United States Congress. I left Congress because I came down with Lyme disease from a tick bite I received while fishing at Quantico Marine Base during a Congressional recess.

My Lyme disease was cured by a special colostrum from a cow after conventional treatments were not effective for me. This has started me on a life journey of investigating alternative treatments for disease. My wife and I have formed The National Foundation for Alternative Medicine. We are sending teams around the world to visit alternative clinics and practitioners to see if we can document effectiveness of treatment. We are finding science and treatments that we believe will change the way the world looks at and treats health and disease.

The colostrum treatment that cured my Lyme disease was a special colostrum in which the pregnant cow had been injected with killed spirochetes, the germs that cause Lyme disease. The theory is if the cow had actually been infected with this disease, the unborn calf would contract the disease before it was born, and Mother Nature would cause the colostrum to have ingredients to cure the calf. It worked for me.

As more and more people turn to natural health remedies, as I did, a plethora of scientific studies on all types of health supplements has become available to inform us. One of those items is colostrum.

Colostrum is the nutrient-rich liquid all mother cows impart to their suckling calves when they are born, prior to the release of milk. Its role in nurturing new life, including that of humans (breastfeeding moms also produce colostrum for the first few days after birth), is to impart essential nutrients that boost the health of a newborn, as well as to pass on immunities from mother to baby. These immunities protect the newborn's delicate system from the many bacteria and pathogens that exist in their new world.

The same nutrients so important to newborns can also rejuvenate our adult bodies. Once we pass puberty, our bodies gradually produce less of the immune and growth factors that help us fight disease and heal damaged body tissue. The result? Aging. The many nutrients present in bovine colostrum—antibodies, growth hormones, proteins, enzymes, vitamins and minerals—help restore our bodies to the optimum state of our youth. Research has shown that colostrum supplementation increases energy, stimulates tissue repair, kills bacteria and viruses and optimizes cellular reproduction. Cellular reproduction, as well as an abundance of growth hormone, have direct anti-aging effects.

Though science has been able to isolate some of the compounds found in colostrum, their intake can be questionable. For example, when the New England Journal of Medicine reported that growth hormone was the best anti-aging remedy, anti-aging specialists began using it on their patients in earnest. Though recipients reported many anti-aging benefits both external (smoother skin, increased energy and stamina, increased sex drive) and internal (immune system revitalization, organ rejuvenation, and less incidence of osteoporosis), it soon became apparent that there were harmful side effects as well. High blood pressure, the increased growth of unwanted cells in the body (tumors), edema and more turned into reports on the 10 o'clock news as growth hormone therapy came under fire.

Colostrum is a nutritious whole food; the way nature intended it to be. It has been the subject of numerous studies supporting its ability to restore optimum health. We owe a debt of gratitude to the writers and experts of Healthy Living for researching this matter, and for putting it into this easy to read book, so that people can be aware of and informed of this non-toxic food substance. In a special form it has been of great benefit to me—And, as you will see in this book, when properly prepared regular colostrum has been of great help to others.

Berkely Bedell

Former Congressman Bedell was involved with his friend, Senator Tom Harkin, in the establishment of the Office of Alternative Medicine at the National Institutes of Health. With his friend Senator Tom Daschle he wrote The Access to Medical Treatment Act. He is the founder of The National Foundation for Alternative Medicine.

Chapter 1

Colostrum — Timeless Miracle of Birth

Americans are bombarded with messages touting the benefits of drinking milk. In school, on television, and in slick magazine advertisements, we are told that our daily diets are not complete without milk or other forms of dairy products.

But here's a secret: less well known, but possibly of even greater benefit to people's health, is the nutrient-rich product that is first released from mother cow to calf—colostrum.

For many years, the value of colostrum as a healing agent has gone largely unrecognized by the medical and health professions. Today, a plethora of human clinical studies confirm that colostrum is a powerful anti-aging and immune-boosting food that's not just for cows—indeed, it can be used by anyone for better health, increased energy, and longevity. All athletes and fitness buffs will benefit from colostrum's ability to help build lean muscle, repair damaged tissue; and increase energy. Colostrum also helps with specific health problems, helping to perk up an underactive immune system and normalize one that is overactive, as in cases of autoimmune disease (e.g., rheumatoid arthritis, lupus, multiple sclerosis).

Clinical studies on colostrum are one thing—personal success stories are another. The healing stories in this book will put a human face onto colostrum's potential, illustrating how colostrum is a great food for people who want to maintain their health or who are ill and wish to regain their health.

But first things first. Let's answer a few basic questions about what many call "nature's first food."

7

What is colostrum?

Colostrum is a whole food concentrate, replete with thousands of health-promoting, disease-fighting nutrients, many of which haven't even been identified or characterized yet. This is why many experts don't classify colostrum as a dietary supplement—it certainly isn't the same as an herb or an isolated vitamin or mineral. Indeed, it is not considered as a dietary supplement at all, but rather classified by the Food and Drug Administration and other regulatory bodies as simply a food—a very powerful whole food.

What does colostrum contain that makes it so powerful a health aid?

Colostrum is nature's "first food." It is the perfectly balanced "first meal" that every mammal gives its newborn. It is produced by the mother for only a short period of time; yet, it contains numerous compounds that stimulate and support many processes in the body, including activation of the immune system, regeneration and repair of tissues, and growth of all types of cells.

The *immune factors* in colostrum provide protection for the newborn against bacteria, toxins, viruses, and diseases. They activate numerous processes critical to the healthy function of the immune system, and stimulate factors that heighten the overall immune response and provide support to a developing immune system until it is ready to function on its own. These immune factors offer similar benefits to adults and children—stimulating and supporting weakened immune functions while, paradoxically, quieting an overactive immune system.

It's widely known that a mother passes on immunities to her baby through colostrum, and many people are interested in the potential for "passive immunity" from supplemental colostrum. Although there is some immunity passed on from colostrum to the recipient, other remarkable benefits from the immune factors in colostrum come from their ability to strengthen the overall immune response. In the long run, this also has far-reaching health benefits: it means that a weakened immune system can be strengthened to the point where it can ward off invading organisms on its own. This is the ultimate benefit, and the way the immune system was meant to function— without the assistance of donated antibodies via inoculation or otherwise.

Isn't that what we all really want—a healthy immune system capable of taking care of anything that comes along? With healthy immune systems, none of us would have to rely on vaccines and flu shots, which have their drawbacks and are certainly not 100 percent effective. The immune factors in colostrum build and support *all* the processes which relate to healthy immune function. With the regular addition of colostrum to the diet, most individuals report a heightened immune response—fewer colds, flu, and allergies. They also notice that when they do catch a cold, they are able to move through it much more easily.

> Immunoglobulins [found in colostrum] are able to neutralize the most harmful bacteria, viruses, and yeasts.

Growth factors contained in colostrum are instrumental in promoting rapid healing and repair of damaged tissues in the newborn. They are instrumental in facilitating normal growth, and they work with the immune factors to support processes throughout the entire body. For adults and children, these same growth factors are involved in the healing and repair of all types of tissues and organs. With consistent use, they continually regenerate and rebuild the entire body. As with the components of any food, the growth factors in colostrum typically go where they are needed—sealing the lining of the intestinal tract, repairing damaged muscle tissue (including the heart), healing wounds, and rebuilding organs and tissues.

Many of the effects of the growth factors are considered to be anti-aging. The youthful "side effects" of taking colostrum include more

energy, elevated moods, smoother skin, wrinkle reduction, better digestion, balancing of blood sugar levels, and weight loss, to name a few.

How long has bovine colostrum been consumed by humans?

For thousands of years, Ayurvedic physicians and sacred healers
known as Rishis have used bovine (cow) colostrum for medicinal
purposes for everything from immune deficiencies and age-related
symptoms to treatment of the common cold. Even today, colostrum
is delivered with the milk in some parts of India.

In the Scandinavian countries, colostrum has been used in folk
medicine for centuries. The birth of a calf is celebrated and the
colostrum is used in the making of a dessert to promote good health.
As early as 1799, Dr. Hufeland researched the benefits of colostrum
on the health and growth of newborn cattle. His studies laid the
groundwork for the early medicinal use of colostrum.

In the United States, colostrum was used for its antibiotic
properties even before antibiotics were available. In the 1950s,
it became known and respected for its immune-boosting capabilities
and was extensively used in the treatment of rheumatoid arthritis.
In 1962, Albert Sabin developed a successful polio vaccine from
isolated antibodies found in bovine colostrum.

Eventually, the technology that erupted during the aftermath of
World War II produced penicillin and the sulfa drugs. These new
drugs worked so quickly that many traditional methods were
forgotten in favor of faster-working antibiotics.

Now, after 50 years of antibiotic use, we are seeing some serious
drawbacks. Their overuse has caused resistant strains of bacteria
requiring stronger and stronger antibiotics which, in turn, can
trigger unhealthy side effects. Because of this, many people are again
beginning to consider the older, more traditional remedies that were
used for centuries before reliance upon antibiotics and other drugs.

Does colostrum's use go beyond the field of human health?

As with many of the natural remedies now resurfacing, the veterinary industry leads the way. Colostrum has been utilized in the animal industry for many years. A leading authority, Richard Cockrum, D.V.M., of Immuno-Dynamics, Inc., began experimenting with colostrum over 30 years ago. As a young veterinary student, he observed the rapid decline in the health of animals that were deprived of colostrum. His research resulted in the development of a complete line of veterinary colostrum formulations that are still used worldwide—often in place of antibiotics. His work has paved the way in the development of processing methods that ensure safety while retaining the biological activity of the delicate components in colostrum.

Have any scientific studies been published on colostrum's health benefits?

During the last 20 years, the scientific community has rediscovered the multitude of benefits from this natural "food." Over 10,000 experimental and clinical studies have been published on the use of colostrum and its components to treat a variety of diseases and health concerns. In fact, pharmaceutical companies have been so intrigued with many of the components in colostrum that they have synthesized (genetically engineered) several of them, including interferon, protease inhibitors, gamma globulin, growth hormone (GH), and insulin-like growth factor-I (IGF-I). The latter has been used in expensive anti-aging clinics for 10 to 15 years.

How is bovine colostrum obtained?

Bovine colostrum is produced before birth, and can only be collected for a short period of time without being diluted by the subsequent production of milk. At the time of birth, potency is at its peak, with the active elements (immune factors, growth factors, antioxidants, and anti-inflammatory agents) at their highest concentrations. However, in less than 12 hours, the concentration of these components is only half of what it was at the time of birth. This makes colostrum a limited commodity; yet, because of the extensive dairy industry, sufficient quantities are available for human use as a dietary supplement.

Why bovine colostrum?

There are several reasons why bovine colostrum is the chosen source for human supplementation:

- Other than the actual antibodies (specifically produced as a result of contact with pathogens), most of the immune factors and growth factors contained in bovine colostrum have been identified in human colostrum and shown to be very similar. Not only are they very similar; some of the factors in bovine colostrum are many times more potent. For this reason, when it comes to healing and regeneration, bovine colostrum may even be better than human colostrum.

- Bovine colostrum is not species-specific—any mammal can benefit from its use. For this reason, bovine colostrum has been used successfully for many years on a wide variety of animal species. Bovine colostrum is like the universal blood type, "O," which can be utilized by any other blood type.

- Cows produce an abundance of this "first food"—enough to supply human needs without depriving newborn calves. Most cows produce between 2 and 2 1/2 gallons of colostrum from the first milking, but calves only need about two quarts.

- The dairy industry in this country is perfectly suited for the sanitary removal and processing of bovine colostrum. In addition, because the dairy industry is so large, there are plenty of dairy cows from which to "pool" colostrum.

But isn't the newborn calf deprived of an important food for its health?

The first thing most people want to know is: "What happens to the poor calf? Does it have its *first meal* taken away?" Fortunately for everyone, a cow produces more than enough colostrum. If a calf were left to suckle its mother, it would consume only about one of the two quarts of colostrum it typically requires, then lie down to rest. While the calf is sleeping, precious biological factors are reabsorbed back into the mother and lost forever. For this reason, it has been standard practice for many years to remove the colostrum from a mother cow and feed it to the calf from a bottle at intervals so that it can receive the full benefit of this "first milk." Calves actually get more of the benefits of colostrum this way and are healthier with a lower mortality rate.

Research has also shown that there is a point at which calves receive no further benefit from additional colostrum. Two quarts is usually sufficient, unless there are complications. The rest of the colostrum has been used in the veterinary industry for years. Rest assured, no dairy farmer would allow a newborn calf to go without colostrum. In most cases it would mean certain death, since cows rely completely on colostrum for their immunity.

How do cows make colostrum?

Colostrogenesis, which is the formation of colostrum, and *lactogenesis*, the formation of milk, are completely separate processes. They are each controlled by specific hormonal changes and influenced by different physical factors. A common misconception about bovine colostrum is that it continues to be produced after the calf is born.

This is not the case. The hormonal changes that occur at the time of birth cause colostrum production to cease in the mother cow. This is perhaps the *single most important thing* to understand when it comes to colostrum quality.

During the last five to seven years, dairy science has developed a deeper understanding of what bovine colostrum actually is and how it is formed. Numerous studies have now shown that colostrum formation in the cow begins several weeks prior to birth, accelerates as parturition nears, and ceases upon the birth of the calf.

Let's take a closer look at the process:

- The formation of colostrum is initiated in the cow three to four weeks before the birth. At this time, growth factors and other transforming substances are released which influence the appearance of receptors on the lining of the mammary gland. These receptors facilitate the transfer of materials from the mother's blood into the gland.

- Two weeks before birth, these receptors become fully active. Antibodies from the mother's blood known as immunoglobulins attach to the receptors and are transferred into the mammary gland. Additional receptors transport other substances prior to birth.

- About two days before birth, the hormonal balance shifts, initiating the production of secretions and switching on the ability of cells in the mammary tissue to synthesize numerous substances. At the time of birth, the mammary gland is filled with a mixture of immune factors, growth factors, nucleotides, vitamins, enzymes, and minerals which are perfectly balanced to activate and support over 50 processes in the newborn calf.

Is the production of colostrum by humans the same as that in cows?

Colostrogenesis is somewhat different in the human system. A human mother will continue to produce colostrum for about two days. This has caused many to assume that the bovine process is the same. However, bovine colostrum production *ceases* at the time of birth. Hormonal changes associated with birth block any further transfer of substances from the mother's blood into the mammary gland. Therefore, the substance available at the time of birth is the only true colostrum.*

It has a composition characterized by:
1. A high protein content—mostly the Immunoglobulin G (IgG, a class of antibodies).
2. High concentrations of growth promoters.
3. Low lactose concentrations (a milk sugar).
4. Milk fat concentrations between 20 and 30 percent.

How well is bovine colostrum really absorbed into the human body?

While colostrum does contain a large percentage of antibodies, there is some question as to how many of these antibodies are actually able to pass through the adult digestive tract without being broken down. One recent study indicated that between 36 and 68 percent were able to pass through the human system while retaining biological activity. That's a very high percentage, although other estimates indicate that a much smaller amount actually retain their biological activity.

Why do so many health experts talk about first-milking colostrum?

At birth, when the placenta is eliminated, the level of the hormone called progesterone falls dramatically. Simultaneously, a

*See chart "Transition from Colostrum to Normal Milk" on page 18.

protein-based substance develops in the lining of the mammary gland which blocks any further transfer of substances from the mother's blood. These changes, along with the physical removal of the colostrum, signal the production of milk—referred to as lactogenesis.

At the time of birth, almost all of the biologically active components present in the udder are transferred from the circulation of the mother, while most substances found in later fluids are produced by cells within the udder itself. These factors, combined with the time of collection after birth, play a major role in establishing the quality of bovine colostrum. Removal of even a small quantity of colostrum immediately after birth, as would occur via suckling, results in a very substantial influx of a different fluid produced by the cells in the udder, known as transitional milk, markedly diluting the true colostrum.

> As we age, we notice it takes us a little longer to fight off a cold or flu, something aches, our energy and enthusiasm have lessened, our skin loses its elasticity. Aging, illness and death occur with the loss of immune and growth factors in our bodies. Medical science has shown in hundreds of published reports worldwide that these can possibly be replaced in the human body with bovine colostrum.

It is difficult to determine where to draw the line between true colostrum and what has been called transitional milk. At what point in time is colostrum no longer pure colostrum? As veterinary doctor Donald Lein, director of the Veterinary Diagnostic Laboratory at Cornell University, notes:

"Bovine colostrum is produced during the few weeks prior to birth of the calf and, due to hormonal changes in the mother, its production stops at birth. Secretions collected at the first milking during the first 12-hour period after birth contain complete colostrum with all of the beneficial components intact. Removal of even some of the colostrum results in the release of a different material, known as transitional milk, that dilutes any colostrum still present and changes its composition."

In addition, if the true colostrum is not removed from the udder during the first 8 to 12 hours after the birth of the calf, the mother's system begins to reabsorb the biologically active components back into her circulation. Therefore, the only colostrum that contains all of the biologically active components in the appropriate proportions is that which is obtained at the first milking within 12 hours after birth. Major American dairy producers are keenly aware of this and maintain maternity wards separate from the main herd to support the birth of their calves. They no longer allow the calf to suckle but, rather, collect the complete colostrum within hours after birth and feed an adequate quantity to the calf via a nursing bottle.

The removal of even small amounts of colostrum triggers the production of a significant quantity of milk. If colostrum is not removed, or is only partially removed, the mother's system will begin to reabsorb many of the biologically active substances within six to eight hours. This is why most dairy farmers "milk" the cow and feed the required amount back to the calf.

For those of us interested in the best quality colostrum, the *first milking* is the only time it can be obtained in an undiluted state and before biological factors begin to be reabsorbed into the mother. This assures that it is still high in the immune and growth factors most beneficial to health.

Misunderstanding the shift from production of colostrum to production of milk has caused many to believe that good quality colostrum can be produced and collected from the first five milkings of the cow. This is not the case, as the 80/20 rule illustrates.

The 80/20 rule is an accepted concept in dairy science. It refers to the fact that when a cow is milked, no more than 80 percent of the contents of the mammary glands can be removed without damage to the cow. This being the case, the *first milking* of the cow after she gives birth contains 80 percent of the total colostrum which has been produced. The first-milking is a true, undiluted colostrum. Any subsequent milking contains less and less of the total colostrum. For example, the second milking contains 80 percent of the 20 percent which was not removed during the first milking (or about 16 percent of the total colostrum). Even though this second milking contains 16 percent colostrum, it is in a highly diluted state. The third milking contains 80 percent of the remaining 20 percent (or about 3 percent of the total colostrum). Any "colostrum" which is collected after the second milking is in such a diluted state that it can hardly be called colostrum, and in the dairy industry is referred to as *transitional milk*.

This is very important. Too many so-called colostrum products being peddled today are not colostrum but rather transitional milk. Because of this, many consumers who have purchased colostrum seeking to obtain the same healing powers documented in clinical studies have come away disappointed with their colostrum experience. Chapter 3 will show shoppers how to be savvy colostrum consumers.

TRANSITION FROM COLOSTRUM TO NORMAL MILK
dried bovine colostrum

HOURS AFTER	TOTAL				
Calving	Protein	Casein	Albumin	Fat	Lactose
0	65.10	18.82	42.02	18.90	8.11
6	48.90	17.16	30.79	33.48	13.25
12	41.64	20.65	20.37	26.15	25.53
24	35.40	21.61	11.59	26.62	31.17
48	32.64	22.95	8.64	24.43	34.64
72	32.55	22.77	8.18	26.14	36.85

Information from *Fundamentals of Dairy Chemistry*, B.H. Webb, A.H. Johnson & J.A. Alford (eds.). Westport, CT: AVI Publishing, 1978.

To make this point a little more emphatic, take a look at this information from a standard dairy industry text.

Note how fast the total protein fraction of colostrum drops. Within hours, the total protein content is dramatically reduced and within three days is only half of what it was upon birth. This is significant because a good portion of the biological factors which are of interest in colostrum are large protein molecules. The rapid drop in this fraction is indicative of the transition to milk. Also note the rapid increase in lactose, which increases by more than fourfold. This is another very good indicator of the presence of milk.

Since colostrum is a limited commodity, it is easy to see why anyone would want to stretch the collection of this valuable substance. This is why many widely advertised colostrum products on the market today *are obtained from the first five milkings—as much as 72 hours following the birth of the calf.* Such products, although widely sold and labeled as colostrum, are not a true or complete colostrum. Better labeling requirements are necessary to aid shoppers to make smart choices about their nutritional supplements, including colostrum.

It is worth noting that researchers who use colostrum in clinical trials usually seek first-milking colostrum because they recognize that potency and quality are diminished with time. Much of the research referenced in this book, as well as all of the clinical reports and anecdotes, are based on use of first-milking colostrum. To expect similar results with adulterated colostrum or transitional milk being marketed as colostrum would be unfair to both consumers seeking the health benefits of colostrum and to those producers of true first-milking colostrum.

What are the similarities and differences between human and bovine colostrum?

The majority of human immunity is transferred through the placenta. Babies are born with a certain amount of immunity—colostrum is desirable but not absolutely necessary for a baby's survival. Cows receive *no* immunity through the placenta and their immune system is *completely dependent* upon the receipt of colostrum immediately after birth. For this reason, the concentration of antibodies/immunoglobulins is much higher in bovine than in human colostrum. A 1979 study revealed that the immunoglobulin portion of bovine colostrum is 86 percent IgG—the most important immunoglobulin in the body. Human colostrum contains only two percent IgG.

Other biological factors are also more concentrated in bovine colostrum. For example, bovine colostrum has a higher concentration of growth factors. These growth factors (mainly IGF-I and GH) are involved in repair and rejuvenation in the human system. The higher growth factor concentration in bovine colostrum is ideal for building lean muscle, repairing tissues damaged due to age or injury, balancing blood sugar levels, reducing wrinkles, and increasing energy, among many other benefits. For the adult seeking healing, muscle tone, rejuvenation and/or anti-aging effects, bovine colostrum is even more promising than human colostrum would be—if it were even an option.

Although complete identity is an overstatement, bovine colostrum contains many very similar components which appear to benefit the human body in the same way as components in human colostrum. For example, the important growth factor found in bovine colostrum, IGF-I, contains the identical amino acid sequence as human colostrum except for a short segment on the front of the bovine molecule. This segment gets split off during digestion in the stomach, leaving an identical version of the human molecule. Other important biological factors are either identical or so similar that they function in a like manner.

The next chapter will explore more of colostrum's benefits, as well as the true stories of people whose health has flourished with its use.

Chapter 2

Colostrum, The Perfect "Food"

Before birth, a baby is completely dependent upon its mother for its health and well-being. Not only does the developing baby receive nutrients from the mother; the mother's immune system protects it from developing infection as well. A mother and baby are like one during the gestational period, with the baby providing none of its own immunities. (In fact, if it did begin manufacturing its own antibodies, the mother's immune system would detect the presence of a foreign body and begin to attack it!)

But what happens when a baby is born and is suddenly deprived of the immune support it has enjoyed from its mother? Nature provides yet another miracle: colostrum.

Since babies receive antibodies through the placenta, they are born with a certain amount of immunity. Yet, even though a baby receives antibodies from the mother before birth, its immune system is not fully developed until several years later. A newborn is therefore subject to an onslaught of bacterial and viral pathogens within minutes after birth. Immunoglobulins (antibodies) that have been transferred from the mother provide immediate passive support, but they are not sufficient to activate or condition the newborn system to function at full capacity.

Colostrum provides the important substances that begin this process. Ideally, immunoglobulins continue to be passed to the newborn baby in breast milk during the first several years of a baby's life.

This is one of the reasons why breastfeeding is so important. Not only does it continue to provide antibodies, but it contains some of the substances found in colostrum which condition the immune system and prepare it to function on its own. Years of research have shown us that babies who are breastfed have many fewer illnesses and many fewer digestive problems than those who are fed infant formulas. Breastfed babies are less likely to experience diarrhea, ear infections, hospitalization—even sudden infant death syndrome.

Colostrum is the perfect combination of all these necessary immune and growth factors. In fact, these components are not naturally found anywhere else in such high concentrations. The immune factors (including immunoglobulins, leukocytes, lactoferrin, lysozymes, cytokines, and other immune-enhancing substances) protect the newborn from pathogens while they activate or "jump-start" the immune system.

Other components in colostrum stimulate growth and promote rapid healing. This is extremely important considering the ordeal of birth and the injuries it can sometimes cause.

Breastfeeding & Colostrum

The greatest gift a mother can give her baby is its first meal. More and more, we are discovering the benefits of breastfeeding. Beyond the emotional and physical bonding that occurs, we continue to uncover new physiological benefits for mother and child:

- Mother's milk is easier to digest than infant formula. The ingredients in mother's milk are easily assimilated, and they are accompanied with enzymes and cofactors that aid digestion and absorption. Consequently, breastfed babies experience fewer digestive difficulties. They are less likely to have colic, and sometimes—but not always—may be a little less fussy. They are even less likely to become overweight.

- Babies who are breastfed have fewer allergies, including eczema and upper respiratory allergies; they are generally healthier and stronger.

- Breastfed babies have higher IQs than those who are fed formula. In school, they tend to learn faster and have fewer adjustment problems than those who were formula fed.

Mothers who breastfeed have a lower risk of female cancers and osteoporosis. With all these benefits, there is obviously much more to colostrum and breast milk than we are currently capable of understanding or manufacturing. This most precious gift from mother to child begins with colostrum, activating and supporting condition-ing and healing where necessary. Now, children and adults can benefit from its balancing, rejuvenating, and healing benefits as well. Not only is colostrum the perfect food for newborn babies; it is also the perfect supplemental food for many adults and children.

Colostrum for Children

For all children—but especially those who were not breastfed—colostrum can be remarkable. Its immune-supporting properties help children in a variety of ways. Often, the combination of synergistic substances in colostrum is enough to boost immunity and clear chronic infections. The components in colostrum contribute to a more rapid healing and provide support against re-infection.

Children suffering from constant runny noses or chronic infections are some of the ones who can benefit the most from the overall support that colostrum provides as it strengthens the entire immune system. Most parents of children with these kinds of problems notice that, with continued use, the frequency and intensity of colds and flus diminishes.

For children with allergies, parents will find that symptoms are less intense within several months of taking colostrum. Often, allergies clear up entirely.

How can all this be? The components of colostrum have so many balancing effects upon the body that taking it can lessen the severity of many conditions and provide support for superior natural health. Because children have a tendency to respond quickly, the addition of supplemental colostrum to their diets can often make a dramatic difference.

The Howell family of Westover, Penn. discovered this when their 8-year-old niece was diagnosed with juvenile diabetes. "At first we got really scared because her blood sugar went up, but we had been told blood sugar levels might fluctuate while the body was finding a new balance, so we kept giving her the colostrum," Mrs. Howell says. "Within a short period of time, there was marked improvement and insulin levels were reduced. After three months there was no insulin requirement at all—none!"

The Griffith family of Beacon Falls, Conn. watched as their two boys with Duchenne muscular dystrophy benefited from colostrum. When the youngest son began walking on his toes, doctors said he was only several months away from undergoing a procedure called "heel cord lengthening" that his older brother had to have. "We decided to give our boys each two capsules of colostrum a day," says John Griffith. "Several months later, when we visited the doctor again, my son was so much improved that the surgery was not necessary—at least not now. We have continued to give these boys colostrum every day, and even the doctors are impressed with their progress. During our latest visit, the doctor asked them to run down the hall and as they did, he watched in amazement. Their coordination was much improved, and my younger son no longer walks on his toes the way he did." These are just two of the wonderful true healing stories that show how quickly children respond to healing influences. Their bodies utilize healing energy so well that they often bounce back very rapidly when given appropriate support.

Colostrum for Adult Immune Support

Adults who take colostrum do so for many different reasons. Many of them notice positive improvements in other areas of their health as well—a result of the overall natural health boost colostrum provides.

Immune function is just one of the many things that declines with age, and many adults take colostrum for this reason. After taking colostrum for an extended period of time, many people notice that colds and flus are fewer and further between and are less severe when they do come. Many also notice that allergies lessen in severity or disappear altogether.

Why? One reason could be that the growth factors in colostrum have been shown to rejuvenate and aid regrowth in the adult thymus gland, which is central to the healthy function of the immune system. The thymus shrinks in size after puberty until, by the time an individual has reached old age, all that remains are bits of connective tissue. Since the thymus is such an integral part of the immune system, its regrowth has tremendous implications for a healthy immune system.

In addition, several of the many immune factors contained in colostrum are active in fighting off bacteria and viral pathogens:

- *Leukocytes* (white blood cells) actively fight invading organisms, engulfing them using a process known as phagocytosis. They also play an important role in removing the toxins left by harmful organisms.

- *Lactoferrin* is an iron-binding protein with numerous immune-enhancing properties, including antimicrobial as well as antiviral activities. Its ability to bind iron keeps many bacterial infections from spreading because the organisms lack the iron necessary to replicate.

- Several enzymes, including *lysozymes* and *peroxidase*, are active in breaking up and hydrolyzing bacteria.

- *Oligo-polysaccharides* and *glycoconjugates* attract and bind to pathogens, preventing them from attaching to host sites in the digestive tract.

The above are components with *active* roles in fighting harmful organisms. Still other immune factors found in colostrum have regulatory or interactive roles, enhancing or suppressing the production of killer cells, T-cells, interferon, and other important substances involved in healthy immune function. Colostrum helps wherever it's needed, boosting both overactive and depressed immune systems.

Take the case of Janine O. of Riverside, Calif., who was diagnosed with adult asthma brought on by allergies several years ago. After taking colostrum, she no longer had to call in sick to work. "Since I have been taking 'first-milking' colostrum, I can honestly say I have not had one allergy attack," she says. "I have also felt better and had more energy."

Burning Fat and Building Muscle with Colostrum

Weight loss is often an unintended but welcome surprise for people taking colostrum. Two of the growth factors in colostrum, notably growth hormone (GH) and Insulinlike Growth Factor-I (IGF-I), play a significant role in the body's ability to burn fat and build lean muscle.

A report from the University Clinic of Internal Medicine in Denmark concluded that GH prevents the body from burning glucose for energy and instead increases fat oxidation. GH also acts as a catalyst in the production of IGF-I, which is involved in nutrient uptake and the growth of muscle cells. Tests conducted on elderly Swedish people with low amounts of lean muscle mass and lost strength and exercise capacity noted distinct improvement when participants received GH supplements. It was also observed that even though muscle mass increased, overall weight did *not*, indicating that fat was burned while muscle was gained.

As it turns out, the interactive influence of both GH and IGF-I has a major influence on metabolism. Together, GH and IGF-I restore many important metabolic processes in the aging body. This often results in a decrease in body fat and a shift from fat to lean muscle tissue.

"[When I started taking colostrum] I didn't realize it would help me lose weight, but I have been able to lose 20 pounds during the last three months without changing my diet," says Pete D. of Colorado Springs, Colo. "I used to play football in college but ever since I quit, I have put on a little more weight each year. Three months ago, I weighed 250 pounds. Now I am down to 230—without even trying."

"I took about 11,000 milligrams of first-milking colostrum per day for several months before reducing to a lesser amount," adds Janet W. of Anaheim, Calif. "I have had some marvelous success with slimming down. I have lost inches without altering my diet."

Increased Energy

Another interesting benefit that many individuals using colostrum discover is increased energy. For many, it is almost immediate. It is hard to pinpoint the exact reason why colostrum increases energy;

there are undoubtedly several. Because colostrum helps balance many functions and processes in true holistic fashion, it is safe to assume that the energy which would have been expended in these areas is now available for other things. Colostrum also significantly aids the digestive process, which enhances nutrient uptake and utilization. This alone could account for the additional energy many experience.

"I have energy that I haven't had in years," says colostrum user Judy D. of Phoenix, Ariz. "I am in my forties, but I really feel like I did when I was in my twenties!"

"When I began taking colostrum, I initially felt very sick," comments Jill S. of Auburn, Wash. "I got a fever and was more tired for a couple of days. Then, I got my strength back, and I felt more energy than I had felt in three years. The aches and pains subsided, and the perpetual sore throat went away."

Another user had a long-standing iron deficiency corrected with colostrum. "I struggled with anemia long before I realized what it was," says Leanne W. of Berkeley, Calif. "I have done many things to try and help my body absorb iron because supplementation alone did not seem to do the trick."

"I found out about 'first-milking' colostrum and began taking 1,000 mg a day. Now, eight months later, my blood tests are all in the normal range—finally. My energy level is balanced and I feel good, no more exhausting fatigue. The only change I made was adding colostrum . . . in fact, a lot of days I missed taking my iron. This is the best news I've had in years!"

Healing & Rejuvenation

The growth factors in colostrum provide the means for healing and regeneration throughout the entire body.

One of the first places colostrum "goes" is to the lining of the intestines. This is where many illnesses actually begin. The lining of the intestines is under constant assault from toxins, microorganisms, refined foods, food preservatives, chemicals, and antibiotics. Damage in this area allows invaders such as pathogens, allergens, toxins, and undigested food into the bloodstream, where they can cause serious consequences. The growth factors in colostrum help to seal the lining of the whole digestive tract, reducing inflammation and closing the "holes" caused by these invaders. As a result, ulcers heal, allergies improve, nutrient absorption improves, and the line of defense against pathogens returns to more normal function.

Just as the growth factors in colostrum are able to rejuvenate the thymus gland, they have also been shown to bring new vitality and healthy cell growth to heart and lung tissue. Their regenerative benefits are responsible for the repair of tissues throughout the body including skin, muscle, cartilage, and bone. A 1981 study identified seven different growth promoters in colostrum involved in both growth and repair of body cells. Three of these are involved in the healing of wounds.

Colostrum helped heal the wounds of Dallas S. of Aberdeen, Wash. "I had an open ulcer on my leg about the size of a silver dollar for four years," he says. "Doctors treated me for four months without success. For the next four years, I tried everything that came my way, from healing salves and lotions to chlorophyll compounds. Nothing made very much difference, until I found out about colostrum."

Dallas began making a thick paste using three or four capsules of colostrum mixed with oxygenated water. He spread this on his wound every morning and evening, and ingested eight capsules per day as well.

"Within a month there was noticeable improvement, and in just two months, all that remained of the original ulcer was a small scab and very pink skin in the area where the ulcer had been," Dallas remembers gratefully.

Finally, Arland R. of Mountain View, Calif., says colostrum helped with her heart problems. "I was diagnosed with congestive heart failure," she says. "I was told that I had an enlarged heart and that there was a certain percentage of it that was actually 'dead.' My doctor told me he had never seen a heart muscle rebuild from that kind of damage."

The doctor told Arland that she would have to severely limit her physical exercise for the rest of her life. But that was before she started taking colostrum.

"I recently had a number of tests, including an echo cardiogram, X-rays, and an EKG," Arland happily reports. "After one year of taking colostrum, tests showed that my heart was back to normal size—and now my doctor says that one of the best things I could do was exercise."

Anti-aging

It is now well-documented that the hormones in the body decrease as we age. One of the key hormones is, again, GH. Several studies indicate that advanced age is associated with reduced levels of GH and its counterpart, IGF-I. It has been reported that by the age of 40, the concentration of IGF-I is less than half of what it was at age 20.

Likewise, GH decreases about 80 percent between the ages of 21 and 61. Hormone reductions cause the skin to thin and dry out, muscle mass and bone density to decrease, cholesterol levels to rise, cardiovascular function to weaken, and mental abilities to decline.

In a landmark study in the *New England Journal of Medicine*, six months of GH treatment not only stopped the body from aging, but actually reversed the effects of years of hormone deficiency. This study, conducted with 26 men between the ages of 61 and 80, resulted in an overall decrease in body fat (up to 14 percent), an increase in lean muscle mass, and thicker, more elastic skin.

The study equated these changes with the reversal of 10 to 20 years of aging!

Subsequently, genetically engineered hormone replacement has become more popular. Growth hormones, it seems, are being used on an increasing basis to prevent aging.

However, colostrum supplementation may be a more viable and desirable option. The more we learn about the body, the more we understand that no function is completely independent. Furnishing a "whole food" is usually much preferred over supplying portions in isolation. Colostrum is a balanced and complete "food" and is 100 percent natural. It contains all the hormones used by the body—not just one—and in appropriate proportions. These growth hormones are accompanied with all the factors and co-factors needed to work together for maximum benefit. There are no side effects, and thousands of years of use have proved there are no complications.

Besides having more energy, those who use colostrum regularly report that they "just feel better." GH affects neurotransmitters in the brain, improving mood and enhancing mental functions and memory.

"I have noticed that my outlook on life is more positive," writes colostrum user Ronald O. of Mt. Hood, Oregon.

"After two years of taking colostrum, I ran into a friend I hadn't seen in a couple of years," says Mary P. of Hamilton, N.Y. "The following week he called me and asked me what I had been doing to look so young. He said I looked 10 years younger than when he had seen me last—that my skin was visibly different."

To produce the anti-aging benefits seen in people like Mary, the growth factors in colostrum stimulate cell growth in the dermal layer of the skin, improving both skin thickness and elasticity.

In this way, wrinkles are reduced and the skin takes on a soft texture.

Cell proliferation is also stimulated in the scalp, and some colostrum users, like Dorothy H. of West Hills, Calif., have even seen hair regrowth. "I decided to make a topical formula for my skin," says Dorothy. "I mixed colostrum with extra virgin olive oil and put it on my face at night. Believe it or not, there is hair growing from the places in my hairline where it had begun to get thin."

"I have a lot of patients who love colostrum for the anti-aging effects," says chiropractor/holistic doctor Greg Barsten. "I treated a naturopath recently for low energy by using colostrum. Not only did her energy pick up, but her husband (an engineer of the skeptical nature) came to me wanting some. 'Just look at her face—the wrinkles are gone!' he said. I have had several people come to me asking for colostrum because of what it has done for their friends."

Colostrum is used as a supplement by so many people with so many beneficial effects—no wonder people call it the "perfect food."

Chapter 3

Colostrum—What's in it?

Now that you have an insight into bovine colostrum and what complete first-milking colostrum really is, take a look at what it is composed of.

The Basic Composition of Colostrum: Proteins

Complete first-milking bovine colostrum is a thick, golden-colored fluid that contains many proteins, many of which are biologically active. Of all the healing substances found in colostrum, proteins convey the most significant health benefits. Since almost all of the beneficial proteins are conveyed from the mother's bloodstream into the colostrum before birth and the mother then begins to reabsorb them about six to eight hours after birth, it is important to use first-milking colostrum.

A number of scientific studies have validated the superior nutritional value of first-milking colostrum taken within six to eight hours after birth. By 24 hours after birth, most of the proteins in the udder fluid consist of two individual proteins that are primarily only of nutritional value: casein, which is available in ordinary milk products, and albumin, which is similar to the albumin found in egg whites.

The proteins in first-milking colostrum are manufactured from various amino acids and carry out numerous functions within the body. Dried bovine colostrum from the first-milking is 50 to 60 percent protein, of which 30 to 40 percent is immunoglobulins. The remainder of the protein fraction is composed of casein, albumin, and various immune modulating and growth promoting substances. Therefore, good quality complete first-milking colostrum should contain 45 to 60 percent protein, of which about 30 to 40 percent will be immunoglobulins.

Fats

Many colostrum products on the market today have been de-fatted. In a culture that worships "nonfat" and "low-fat" products, most people don't realize that this compromises the effectiveness of the product.

When it comes to colostrum, fat is a good thing. De-fatting colostrum compromises the overall effectiveness and leads to the disappearance of many valuable components that are closely associated with the fat molecule.

Milk fat is one of the most underrated and misunderstood components in complete first-milking colostrum. Many companies that promote bovine colostrum for human consumption have disseminated stories, none of which are substantiated with any scientific evidence, that the fat in colostrum doesn't serve any purpose and/or that having it there leads to faster deterioration of the product. Nothing could be further from the truth! In fact, one company that removes fat from what they call "colostrum" adds a component of the fat back to their dried products. They claim that this makes their "colostrum" more digestible, which was one of the functions of the fat in complete colostrum in the first place.

Mother nature doesn't waste and has organized the components of colostrum in an efficient way to maximize its benefits for offspring. High quality first-milking bovine colostrum will contain 20 to 30 percent milk fat, and milk fat in colostrum is a very important means to deliver some of its beneficial biologically active substances. Dissolved in or associated with the fat in colostrum are the following substances:

- Fat-soluble vitamins (A, D, E, and K).
- The valuable growth factor known as IGF-I.
- Additional growth factors.
- Steroid hormones.
- Corticosteroids.
- Insulin, which is related to the growth hormone, IGF-I.

When we refine foods, we take ingredients out—only to later have to "fortify" the food in order to return at least some of its nutritional value. But as hard as we try, fortification can never match the original balance in a "whole" food. The same is true with colostrum. When the makers of colostrum products on the market today de-fat their products and/or add milk lipid (fat) molecules back into the product after de-fatting, the effectiveness of this delicately balanced food is compromised.

De-fatting removes approximately 35 percent of the highly prized growth factor, IGF-I. This can mean a significant reduction in colostrum's anti-aging effects, muscle building capacity, energy value, and, especially, its ability to repair damaged tissues. De-fatting also removes large portions of the fat-soluble vitamins A, D, E, and K, and other growth promoters.

Studies have also shown that milk fat plays an extremely important role during the processing of colostrum, protecting the antibodies and proteins that are sensitive to heat during pasteurization and drying. Pasteurization of a de-fatted, first-milking colostrum reduces the biological activity of antibodies by 50 percent. But if the fat is left intact, there is only a five percent loss of biological activity.

Years of experience have taught many of us the importance of whole foods. Colostrum is no different. It is a "food" and, as such, is a perfectly natural source of ingredients that are designed to work together to balance, repair, nourish, and revitalize the body. Changes or amendments disrupt this balance and impair its ability to function as a "whole" food.

Lactose (Milk Sugar)

Lactose is the sugar in milk that some adults cannot completely digest. A good quality first-milking colostrum contains a lower lactose level than transitional milk—between 10 and 15 percent.

After about age four, some people gradually lose lactase, the enzyme that is responsible for the digestion of lactose. Without it, lactose cannot be broken down into simple sugars that the body can use. For these adults, known as "lactose intolerant," the ingestion of milk products causes cramps, bloating, gas or other allergic reactions.

Certain ethnic groups have a higher tendency toward lactose intolerance than others. People of Asian and African American descent generally have a higher incidence of lactose intolerance than do Caucasian peoples, for example. However, even 10 percent of the Caucasian race is lactose intolerant.

Levels of lactose in colostrum increase rapidly during the first few hours after birth—doubling in less than 12 hours. This means that if colostrum is taken from the cow after 12 hours, it may cause an allergic response in those with lactose intolerance. Lactose intolerant individuals can usually handle about 75 milligrams of lactose—about two bites of a cheese pizza. This is why many manufacturers of colostrum add lactase to their product. However, this isn't usually necessary with first-milking colostrum, in which levels of lactose are usually low enough so that even lactose intolerant individuals can safely benefit.

Severely lactose intolerant individuals who want to take colostrum might consider taking the enzyme lactase (available in most health food stores) along with their colostrum supplements; however, in general, first-milking colostrum should be safe even for lactose intolerant people. Indeed, many allergies fade away with the continued use of first-milking colostrum—even the allergic reaction to milk products. After using first-milking colostrum, many individuals find that they can tolerate milk as well as other foods that previously caused them difficulty.

Moisture Removal
Good quality colostrum is carefully spray dried at a low temperature to remove the moisture, which increases its shelf life and reduces degradation. With a moisture content of under six percent, the shelf life is likely to exceed three years, regardless of whether or not the fat has been removed.

These four factors are important markers in identifying a good quality colostrum. If any of the above is disproportionate, it is an indicator that the product is either not true colostrum or that it has been denatured in some way. In either case, it is not likely to be as effective as a whole, first-milking colostrum.

Did You Know? Colostrum vs. Milk
The following comparative facts about colostrum and milk further stress the need to use complete first-milking colostrum in order to maximize the benefits that it can provide:

- Colostrum contains 10 times more vitamin A than milk.
- Colostrum contains 3 times more vitamin D than milk.
- Colostrum contains at least 10 times more iron than milk.
- Colostrum contains more calcium, phosphorous, and magnesium than milk.

Colostrum: Individual Components and What They Do
To date, over 80 different components have been isolated from

colostrum. These components work together synergistically to produce the profound healing, health maintenance, and rejuvenation miracles that only colostrum can provide.

The biologically active components in complete first-milking colostrum can be divided into categories based upon the health aspect where they exert their greatest influence. As we go through the discussion of what these substances do, you will see that in some cases the functions of these components can be clearly separated into categories, while in other cases, the dividing line is not as clear.

The major categories are the Immune Factors (Immune Helpers), Growth Factors (Tissue Repair Helpers), and Metabolic Factors.

Immune Helpers

- **Immunoglobulins**, also called antibodies, neutralize invading pathogens in the lymphatic and circulatory systems. Many people take colostrum for the immunoglobulins (Ig) in an effort to receive immunity for a wide range of pathogens. Thanks to its immunoglobulins, colostrum consistently has an effect on pathogens that invade the intestinal tract causing diarrhea and gastrointestinal illness.

- **Leukocytes** are living white blood cells that play an important role in fighting infection and in clearing toxins left by invading organisms. Colostrum contains several different kinds of leukocytes, including lymphocytes, macrophages and phago-cytes that engulf and destroy viral and bacterial organisms. Leukocytes also stimulate the production of other immune factors, including interferon, which "interferes" with the reproduction of viruses.

- **Lactoferrin** is an iron-binding protein that aids the body in utilizing iron. The ability of lactoferrin to bind iron is important in keeping invading bacteria in check, since they require iron to multiply. Many other functions have been attributed to lactoferrin, including antimicrobial and antiviral activities, immune regulation, and cell-growth regulation. Lactoferrin enhances phagocytosis (the engulfing of harmful organisms by white blood cells) and plays a powerful role in reducing the inflammation that accompanies many health problems.

• **Transferrin** is yet another mineral-binding carrier protein that attaches to available iron. It can act independently or in concert with lactoferrin to impede the growth of certain aerobic bacteria, particularly in the gut.

• **Lysozyme** is an enzyme found naturally in colostrum, egg white, saliva, human tears, and blood. Its natural function is to attack bacteria foreign to the body. Any bacteria invading the body through typical routes such as the eyes, mouth, nose or a cut will meet with the human immunological system, of which lysozyme is a critical part.

Biologically, lysozyme attacks the cell wall of certain bacteria. By nicking the cell in numerous spots, lysozyme gradually weakens the wall. When the osmotic pressure within the cell is too much for the weakened wall to withstand, the bacterium will burst.

Lysozyme is so important that it has recently been added to some baby formulas. It has already gained huge popularity in Europe and Asia. Its anti-infectious activity is well touted in the Asian pharmacological industry; in Korea and Japan, pharmaceutical tablets and capsules containing this egg-white derived protein are sold.

- **Peroxidase** is an enzyme that generates the release of hydrogen peroxide to "burn" or hydrolyze bacteria.

- **Proline-rich polypeptide** (PRP) is a small protein chain in colostrum with the same ability to regulate the immune system as the hormones of the thymus gland, as reported by a 1979 study published in *Immunology*.

   PRP helps regulate the immune system to maintain balance between under- and over-activity—extremely important for those with autoimmune disease. It is also a very powerful anti-inflammatory agent, which may help relieve painful flair-ups. Proline-rich polypeptide also stimulates the body's immune cells to produce cytokines: immune-regulating proteins that regulate the duration and intensity of the body's immune response.

In a 1998 study conducted at the Laboratory of Virology, Institute of Immunology and Experimental Therapy, Polish Academy of Sciences, Wroclaw, Poland, it was shown that when proline-rich polypeptide isolated from bovine colostrum was added to the immune cells found in the membrane lining the abdominal cavity and viscera immediately after virus absorption or one day before or after viral infection, infected cells were better able to inhibit virus replication.

This is critically important: immune cells found in the gastrointestinal tract produce about 75 percent of the antibodies in the body. Since colostrum stimulates the immune cells in the gastrointestinal tract, it has great potential to support strong and protective immune function.

- **Cytokines** have a broad influence and are involved in the production of T-cells, lymph activity, and in regulating the force and duration of your body's immune response. One cytokine, known as interleukin-10, is highly anti-inflammatory and a key helper in relieving discomfort among persons with arthritis-related joint pain.

- **Lymphokines** are hormone-like peptides released by activated white blood cells. Lymphokines help to regulate the immune response.

- **Oligosaccharides** and **glycoconjugates** bind to the surfaces of the intestines, preventing the attachment of pathogens there. Evidence is also available that these components act as growth promoters for the beneficial flora in the gastrointestinal tract.

- **Thymosin** is a hormone composed of two protein-based chains, known as alpha or beta chains. The chains act on the thymus gland independently or in concert with each other to stimulate activation, development, and maintenance of the immune system.

- **Transfer factors** are small proteins produced in response to the body's exposure to certain types of microorganisms, particularly those that reside in deep tissues for a long period of time such as the bacterium that causes tuberculosis. They are specific for a particular microorganism and are carried inside of certain types of specialized white blood cells. Transfer factors work in concert with various white blood cells and other factors in an attempt to keep the microorganisms under control.

- **Nucleotides** and **nucleosides** are important for metabolic functions. They enhance antibody responses and contribute to iron absorption during digestion.

- **Orotic acid** has been shown to prevent hemolytic anemia.

- **Xanthine oxidase** is an enzyme that can attach to the cell walls of certain bacteria, and interfere with the ability of the bacteria to replicate.

Tissue Repair Helpers

- **Growth hormone** (GH) is the single most abundant hormone produced by the body, affecting almost every cell. GH levels are highest during teenage years, falling rapidly thereafter. GH increases metabolism, reduces fat and increases muscle mass. It is involved in the regeneration of heart, lung, and liver tissue, as well as many other organs and tissues throughout the body. GH stimulates protein synthesis, which is critical for the renewal of skin and bones. It is also considered to be an immuno-stimulant because it helps the body produce antibodies, T-cells, and white blood cells. GH even affects neurotransmitters in the brain, improving moods and mental acuity.

- **Insulin-like growth factors** (IGF) I and II belong to a whole family of hormones contained in colostrum called the "GF superfamily." IGF-I is considered to be the most potent of these, functioning like the captain of a ship to trigger the events that activate cell growth and reproduction, protein synthesis, and the release of energy (glucose metabolism). Because it is involved in so many major functions, IGF-I is found in association with almost all the cells in the body. It improves the function of GH to build muscle and burn fat, and aids in regenerating and repairing cartilage. Because IGF-I is a primary factor in the ability of cells to grow and reproduce, it is highly desirable for its many anti-aging and regenerative effects.

- **Epithelial growth factor** stimulates normal skin growth.

- **Transforming growth factors A and B** are helpful in healing wounds and in the synthesis and repair of RNA and DNA.

- **Fibroblast growth factor** stimulates the growth of new blood vessels and contributes to tissue development and wound healing.

- **Platelet-derived growth factor** is involved in the healing of vascular wounds. It is released in conjunction with blood clotting during the healing process.

- **Trypsin inhibitors** and other protease inhibitors help prevent the destruction of immune factors and growth factors by enzymes in the gastrointestinal tract. They also prevent the ulcer-causing bacteria, *H. pylori*, from attaching to the walls of the stomach. In this way, they are instrumental in the healing of gastric ulcers.

Metabolic Factors
- **Leptin** is a small hormone-like protein that can suppress appetite and lead to body weight reduction. Leptin deficiency may be associated with obesity, particularly in diabetic individuals.

- **Insulin** is a hormone required for the effective utilization of glucose (blood sugar) in the body. Insulin initiates the conversion of glucose to glycogen, a high-energy source carbohydrate.

- **Vitamin-binding proteins** act as carriers to deliver B-complex vitamins to the body.

- **Mineral-binding proteins**, especially lactoferrin and transferrin, help in the absorption of copper and help keep invading microorganisms from multiplying. Two carrier proteins that assist in calcium absorption—casein, an abundant source of amino acids for building new protein molecules, and alpha-lactalbumin, which is present in appreciable quantities only in first-milking colostrum—are also present in colostrum.

- **Cyclic adenosine monophosphate** (CAMP) provides the chemical energy necessary to form new protein, carbohydrate, and fat molecules.

- **Enzyme inhibitors**, also known as "permeability factors," are actually small proteins that slow down or inhibit the enzymatic breakdown of proteins. They provide protection to the immune, growth, and metabolic factors as they pass through the digestive tract.

Vitamins and Minerals in Colostrum

- **Vitamin A** promotes healthy skin and bone growth. It is essential for proper vision.

- **Vitamin E** is one of the antioxidant vitamins important in membrane structure, as well as playing a critical role in many other interactive functions throughout the body.

- **Vitamin B12** is essential for the formation of red blood cells and in the maintenance of the nervous system. Deficiencies can cause anemia, fatigue and depression.

- **Calcium** performs essential functions in the skeletal, teeth, muscle and nerve tissues. It is important for blood clotting and balanced blood pressure.

- **Sulfur** is a key factor in many bodily processes. It is critical for maintaining the integrity of connective and structural tissues throughout the body. Bioavailable sulfur is the active ingredient in the recently heralded health product known as MSM (methylsulfonylmethane). It is widely used for its ability to reduce inflammatory pain and improve the condition of hair, skin, and nails.

There are many other substances in colostrum that are present in minute quantities, providing little or no benefit to the humans taking it as a supplement. The two other substances in colostrum that do provide significant benefits are the hormone melatonin, which has a direct effect on the establishment of biological rhythms and proper sleep patterns; and relaxin, a hormone known to directly affect contracted muscles.

Chapter 4

Colostrum and The Immune System
Hunter S.'s Ear Infections

Recently, a doctor conducted a placebo-controlled study in conjunction with a daycare center in Salt Lake City. The purpose was to test whether colostrum strawberry chewables for children could reduce the incidence of infectious disease in such a crowded setting. The study was never completed—all because of a little boy named Hunter S.

Hunter, one of the participants in the study, was constantly sick. By the time he was 18 months old, he lived constantly with two sets of tubes in his ears for drainage due to chronic middle ear infections. He had never slept through the night.

One of Hunter's close relatives was a pediatrician who offered to provide medical care for the child, so health care costs were not a problem. As a result of this well-intentioned relative, Hunter had been given just about every antibiotic known to humankind. Unfortunately, this overuse of antibiotics only served to further weaken his immune function.

Within three days of starting on first-milking colostrum, Hunter was sleeping through the night. Within seven days, the fluid buildup and drainage from his ears, nose, and back of throat had ceased. It was a miracle to Hunter's parents.

But there's more.

Hunter's story was not unique. After two months on the chewable strawberry tablets, the parents of the children receiving only the placebo chewables had begun to notice that the kids in the other group were almost all free from colds, flu, allergies, and other respiratory ailments. They also noticed that the children receiving the colostrum chewables seemed happier and were developing better attention spans and listening skills.

The parents of the children on the placebo tablets wanted to know which children were receiving the real thing, and then demanded their children be given the real chewables. If not, they threatened, they would quit the daycare center. The owner could not bear to lose half her clients, so the study came to an end and all of the kids were put on the strawberry colostrum chewables.

Michael C.'s Toxic Overload

It could be said that hairdresser Michael C. of Concord, Calif., works in a very hazardous occupation. Many studies have shown hairdressers to be at relatively high risk for toxic exposures due to the numerous chemicals used in cosmetic and personal care products.

Take hair dyes, to which hairdressers are chronically exposed. Permanent and semi-permanent colors have long contained a wide range of carcinogenic and mutagenic ingredients and contaminants. These have included and, in some cases, still do contain: diaminotoluene, diaminoanisole, and other phenylenediamine dyes; artificial colors; dioxane, a contaminant in detergents and solvents; nitrosamines formed from detergents with nitrite preservatives or contaminants; and formaldehyde-releasing preservatives.

Temporary dyes and rinses contain metals as well as

petrochemicals, which are carcinogenic. They also contain other poorly tested ingredients, such as formaldehyde-releasing preservatives and nitrosamine precursors.

One of the most widely used phenylenediamine dyes, diaminotoluene was "voluntarily" removed by manufacturers in 1971 to avert proposed regulatory action following findings that it induced liver cancer in rodents. By 1979, it was proven to induce breast cancer in rodents. Unfortunately, diaminotoluene was replaced by a closely related chemical (4-ethoxy-m-phenylene sulfate, 4-EMPD). After a report cautioned that there was no significant difference between the two chemicals in their ability to cause cancer, 4-EMPD was "voluntarily" removed from hair coloring products. In 1994, the Food and Drug Administration admitted, in response to requests under provisions of the Freedom of Information Act, that it had never collected information on the toxicity of 4-EMPD, which is still used in a limited number of hair dye products.

Another phenylenediamine, diaminoanisole, was removed from hair dyes in 1978 after it was also found to induce breast and other cancers in rodents. And in 1986, para-phenylenediamine, the basic phenylenediamine dye in current use in virtually all permanent and semi permanent hair-coloring products, was shown to be carcinogenic to the breast following oxidation with hydrogen peroxide.

In short, permanent and semi-permanent hair dyes, among many other cosmeticformulations, have long been a witches' brew of carcinogens and other types of toxins. Besides their individual carcinogenic effects, there is also the likelihood of interactive synergistic effects.

The association between hair dye use and breast cancer is further supported by evidence on excess breast cancers among cosmetologists and hairdressers. Michael, suffering from a high degree of chemical exposure, was no exception.

"After years of exposure, my immune system had taken a beating," he says. "At one point in my career, I participated with other hairdressers in a study to determine the long-term effects of the chemicals we use."

"I had blood tests, allergy tests, and white cell counts under varying circumstances. In the end, it was determined that I was on toxic overload with very little I could do about it if I continued as a hairdresser."

After becoming ill and missing so many appointments that it was becoming a real problem, some of his colleagues suggested he try colostrum.

"I had a runny nose for about 10 days when I began taking the colostrum, and then things started to clear up and I noticed energy-not a 'speedy' feeling, but real, deep-down energy," he says. "The colostrum has also cleared my lungs, and I can breathe deeply again. Now I run around here at work, and everyone wonders what has happened to me."

Dianne T.'s Chronic Fatigue Syndrome

Dianne T., of Tucson, Ariz., had been suffering from infectious chronic fatigue syndrome for 14 years when she was diagnosed with primary immune deficiency. "I knew that I needed the immunoglobulins that were in colostrum, and I had been trying brand after brand without success," she says. "I was becoming very pessimistic because I knew the immunoglobulins were absolutely necessary for my health."

When she tried a "first-milking" colostrum, she was greatly surprised to experience no asthmatic reactions. Because she is allergic to milk, other brands of colostrum had caused both stomach troubles and asthma for her. "The 'first-milking' colostrum eventually solved the milk allergy almost entirely," she adds. "Seven hours after taking those first capsules I stopped getting worse, and within several days I was back to 'normal.'"

"The colostrum seemed to help even more than another immunoglobulin product I had used," Dianne enthuses. "Also, my digestion, which had been an almost continuous problem for 11 years, is now over 95 percent better than in the past. Many supplements and medications give me a rash; colostrum does not and, applied topically, helps the skin problems caused by the other substances."

"I am not yet totally well, and I am continuing to take other supplements and medications (although I was able to cut back on some)," Dianne says. "I know that the colostrum is an essential part of the improvement I am enjoying, and I feel very grateful."

The Immune System: Your Own National Defense System

The immune system is a lot like a national defense system. It is equipped with a military force made up of very specialized units like the Marines, Navy, Air Force, National Guard, and Army. It has a communication network which is unequaled for rapid information exchange. Although the individual subunits have specialized functions, they work as a team and their purpose is the same—to protect the body from invading organisms that will compromise its health.

This internal defense system, which we call the immune system, is so complex that we are only beginning to understand the full scope of its action. Our fully functional defense system is capable of detecting and destroying all harmful "would be" intruders—from those that cause the common cold to those that cause serious maladies such as pneumonia, cancer, and even heart disease. This system is responsible for removing allergens—anything from undigested food particles to pollen, and it's equipped with a Red Cross unit to help clean up the debris resulting from day to day activity and take care of free radical damage wherever it is in the body. Considering the millions of bacteria, viruses, fungi, parasites, and allergens that we encounter on a daily basis, our internal defense system does an amazing job.

We live in a society where immune deficiency is epidemic. Our immune systems are bombarded 24 hours a day with pollutants in the air, in our drinking water, and in our food. Sugar and refined carbohydrates suppress immune function. Electromagnetic frequencies and stress weaken our defense mechanisms. And beyond this, the excessive use of antibiotics has created resistant strains of bacterial pathogens. It's no wonder immune deficiency is at epidemic proportions.

With all of these factors against us, how can we hope to stay healthy unless we can keep our immune systems functioning at peak performance?

The immune system, like every national defense system, can always benefit from a good secret weapon. Colostrum is that weapon. One of the reasons colostrum has been used so successfully by people with immune system disorders like immune deficiency, multiple sclerosis, rheumatoid arthritis, lupus, scleroderma, chronic fatigue syndrome, and allergies is that it is a particularly rich source of bioactive immune factors that help fine-tune immune function. By affecting both individual components of human immunity and the immune system as a whole, the factors in colostrum work together to provide support for a healthy immune system, supporting, balancing, and even rebuilding some of the immune components for a more fully functional system. In this way, colostrum strengthens all of the troops, helping with the continual battle against invaders of all types.

Many drug manufacturers have tried to isolate and synthesize individual immune factors found in colostrum, including interferon and gamma globulin. But there is no question that for most people, the whole intact immune complement found in colostrum is far superior.

As Zoltan P. Rona, M.D., M.Sc., reported in the March 1998 issue of the *American Journal of Natural Medicine*: "Historically, Ayurvedic physicians have used bovine colostrum therapeutically in India for thousands of years. In the United States and throughout the world, conventional doctors used it for antibiotic purposes prior to the introduction of sulfa drugs and penicillin. In the early 1950s, colostrum was prescribed extensively for the treatment of rheumatoid arthritis. In 1950, Dr. Albert Sabin, the polio vaccine developer, discovered that colostrum contained antibodies against polio and recommended it for children susceptible to catching polio."

Holistic physician Nikki-Marie Welch, M.D., of Sedona, Ariz., uses colostrum both personally and in treating patients. "I consider it an important therapeutic aid for all patients with chronic infections, including bacterial, viral, or fungal. Examples of such infections involve recurrent sinusitis, bronchitis, hepatitis, urinary tract infections, and other bacterial invasions; herpes, Epstein Barr, and additional viral diseases; plus the yeast syndrome, candidiasis.

"I start everyone with acute infections on bovine colostrum," she continues. "But in my experience, the patients who gain the most from it are those with chronic and recurrent disease symptoms such as chronic fatigue syndrome, infectious diarrhea, sinusitis, and fibromyalgia."

Welch, who sees many cases of sinusitis in her part of the country, recommends bovine colostrum as an immune system booster to her patients. And because of her own history of metastatic breast cancer, she takes colostrum as part of her own immune boosting program. "I suggest its use to any patient who needs an immunological pick-up," she says.

Before getting into the specifics of how the components in colostrum help fight disease, it's important to have an understanding of how our bodies ward off illness. Let's take a look at how our personal defense systems protect us from the invaders that wreak havoc on our health.

At the Front Line: Components of the Immune System

Immunity is the body's ability to fight off or resist disease and overcome infection. In the complete absence of the immune system, we would not last more than a few days. Because the task is so huge, the immune system must have a presence throughout the body. Immune cells are everywhere. Additionally, there are certain organs and structures, which are designed to carry out major functions for the immune system, just like we have military installations in varying parts of the country.

- **Bone marrow** In the military, everything begins in boot camp. In our internal defense system, all of the cells that function as part of the immune system (and there are dozens of different kinds) originate in the bone marrow. Besides producing red blood cells and platelets, the bone marrow is constantly putting out new immune recruits from boot camp.

- **Thymus** The thymus is a gland found in the center of the upper chest that serves as a basic training center for new cadets. Through a remarkable maturation process referred to as *thymic education*, immature T-cells migrate from bone marrow to the thymus where they mature. T-cells are eliminated if they show a tendency to cause an autoimmune response. Those that develop the attribute known as "self-tolerance" are released into the bloodstream as fully functional soldiers.

- The major regulating hormone for the thymus is known as **proline-rich polypeptide** (PRP). Without PRP, the thymus would allow too many "uneducated" T-cells into the system, which could potentially cause autoimmune problems. PRP is like a drill sergeant, making sure that soldiers have the skills necessary to protect the terrain without becoming over-aggressive. That colostrum contains PRP may account for its ability to "tone down" an overactive immune system, as in the case of autoimmune diseases.

  The thymus plays a central role in the coordination of immune function. It grows rapidly in young children as the immune system builds and expands its capability. However, after puberty, the thymus gradually diminishes in size. By the time old age sets in, there is usually only a bit of connective tissue left. This is perhaps one reason why immune function decreases with age.

As mentioned earlier, colostrum contains growth factors that have been shown to regrow the thymus gland. Two separate studies have shown that growth factors contained in colostrum were able to regrow the thymus to youthful proportions. This fact has some thought-provoking implications on aging and overall immune function.

- *Lymph nodes* Lymph nodes are small bean-shaped structures that are strategically placed throughout the lymphatic system. They are concentrated in the neck, groin, armpits, upper chest, and abdomen. They have two main functions: one, they act as a filter for the lymph system removing debris and foreign matter, and two, they capture and destroy microorganisms. Indeed, the lymph nodes can be major centers of conflict; invaders are brought here and destroyed and it is often a hot and heavy battleground. This is why lymph nodes have a tendency to swell during infection.

- *Spleen* The spleen acts as a filter for the blood. It contains numerous immune cells that capture harmful organisms in the bloodstream and bring them to the spleen, where "seek and destroy" devices (antibodies) are manufactured.

When an invading organism is brought to the spleen, it is detained before destruction so that attachment sites can be matched. Antibodies are manufactured to have an exact "fit" to the invading organism, just like the pieces of a jigsaw puzzle. This acts like a homing device, seeking out other intruders of the same nature.

The Body's Soldiers: Immune Cells

- *T cells* are lymphocytes, a type of white blood cell that matures in the thymus. They are divided into two major groups: T-helper cells and T-killer/suppressor cells. T-helper cells activate other cells and coordinate regulation of the immune response. T-killer/suppressor cells are involved in directly killing tumor cells and cells infected with virus and parasites. These cells are also involved in the suppression of the immune response when the job is done. Both types of cells are found throughout the body, the most active sites being the lymph nodes and the spleen.

- *Natural Killer (NK)* cells are similar to T-killer cells and have similar functions. However, they outrank T-killer cells. They are able to kill target cells without being "activated" in the lymph nodes or spleen. NK cells target cancerous and viral-infected cells, notably herpes and cytomegalovirus.

- *B cells* are also lymphocytes that produce antibodies in response to foreign proteins, bacteria, and virus and tumor cells. Antibody production is critical as a means of signaling other cells to engulf, kill, and remove harmful substances from the body.

- *Leukocytes* (white blood cells) are divided into several categories. Their major function is to engulf or swallow foreign material in a process called *phagocytosis*. Antigens are then presented to T-cells in order to initiate the immune response, which involves the formation of antibodies and the destruction of the invader.

Macrophages are important in the regulation of the immune response. They are often referred to as "scavengers" and "antigen presenting cells" because they ingest foreign materials and present them to T cells and B cells as a first step in the initiation of the immune response. They play an important role in the cleanup after a conflict, ingesting dead cells and removing them from the body.

FYI: Causes of Immune Suppression

Many factors can suppress the immune system and cause vulnerability to dangerous organisms and disease. Most of these are related to stress in one form or another: emotional discord, financial problems, insufficient sleep, toxic buildup (from cigarette smoke, pesticides, drug residues, industrial chemicals, heavy metals), and antibiotics.

The leukocytic index (LI) is a measurement of the number of organisms which one white blood cell can engulf in an hour. This is a significant method of measuring immune function, since white blood cells are one of the most important factors in protecting us from invaders.

The average LI in the U.S. is 13.9. However, after a person eats a meal high in refined carbohydrates, the LI drops to about 1.4 within 15 minutes. In other words, our immune function is suppressed by over 90 percent when we eat sugar and refined carbohydrates. This ought to be enough to help convince anyone to curb their intake of sugar. Excess sugar and fat intake can suppress the immune system for up to two hours.

Even too little or too much exercise can suppress overall immune function for a period of time. On top of that, when the immune system is additionally stressed by ongoing and low-grade infections such as Candida or sinus infections, it does not have the capacity to fully react to numerous invaders, which are everywhere.

Luckily, the antibodies and immune factors in colostrum help to protect us from the type of infections that cause colds and flu and perhaps even more serious illnesses.

Now let's look at the antibodies / immunoglobulins found in both bovine colostrum and our own bodies that protect against illness.

Breakdown: Immunoglobulins

Antibodies / immunoglobulins are grouped into five main categories: IgA, IgD, IgE, IgG, and IgM. Each of these types of antibodies function in a unique way to fight off invaders:

IgA makes up approximately 15 percent of the total number of antibodies within a human adult. These immunoglobulins are especially effective for enteric (gastrointestinal) organisms.

FIGURE 1.

Composition (mg/100ml) of the Ig Portion of Bovine "First-milking" Colostrum	
IgG	3800
IgA	200
IgM	180
IgD	<10
IgE	<10

IgD and **IgE** are not very plentiful in the human system. IgE makes up only .002 percent of the total Ig in the body; however, it is highly antiviral and antiallergenic, with unique properties against tumors and cancer.

IgG is the most abundant class of antibodies, comprising over 80 percent of the total Ig in the adult human immune system. When colostrum is tested for immunoglobulins, this is the group that is usually measured. In human colostrum the IgG is only two percent of the total, because these immunoglobulins have already been transferred through the placenta. They are found at much higher levels in bovine colostrum.

But don't judge your colostrum based on levels of IgG alone. By concentrating these immunoglobulins, other beneficial immune and growth factors may be removed. The most important thing to look for is a complete first-milking colostrum.

IgM is especially effective against bacterial infections.

Since immunoglobulins are produced as a result of invading organisms or antigens, the immunoglobulins in colostrum are never exactly the same. Each cow is exposed to different organisms and produces different antibodies. Unless the cow is inoculated with known organisms, the resulting antibodies can never be counted on to fight specific pathogens.

In other words, to claim that colostrum is always effective against a certain organism would be an overstatement. Still, certain classes of microorganisms seem to respond to supplemental colostrum on a repeated basis. This may indicate that cows are repeatedly exposed to these same organisms.

Most of us have suppressed immune systems at one time or another due to stress. Anything we can do to reduce the stress is good. On the other hand, some people suffer from chronic immune deficiency. These individuals have such depleted immune function that support measures are sometimes necessary. The use of immunoglobulins for this is still being investigated, but early reports look promising.

Chapter 5

Colostrum vs. Common Causes of Infectious Disease
Bacterial Infections

Because of recent public health outbreaks involving bacteria such as E. Coli and salmonella, a considerable amount of research has been done with colostrum regarding bacterial infections that may affect the intestinal tract. Bacterial pathogens such as E. coli, salmonella, shigella, streptococci, and clostridium are notorious for invading the intestinal lining, causing diarrhea, gastrointestinal distress, and other complications.

Colostrum has a good track record with these types of infections. The cessation of diarrhea and other symptoms is very common after supplementation with colostrum. For this reason, many people either take or increase the amount of colostrum they ingest prior to traveling to avoid complications from bacterial infections. Children's diarrhea may especially benefit from colostrum, according to clinical studies.

Holistic doctor Greg Barsten often advises patients who travel not to forget their colostrum.

"I recommend it for people who travel a lot or who are planning an extended vacation," he says. "Airplanes are notorious for spreading pathogenic organisms because of the recycled air. And sanitation in other countries can sometimes be a problem, so I recommend taking colostrum several days prior to a trip."

CLINICAL CASE REPORT: Lawrence Levy

Lawrence L. of Eureka, Calif., had ulcerative colitis for about four years. During the last year, the diarrhea and bleeding had gotten so bad that he had to go to the bathroom 20 times a day, bleeding every time. Doctors had tried several different medications; none of them worked.

"I was so tired and run down that if I hadn't discovered colostrum, I don't know where I would be today," says Lawrence. "I could tell a difference within two weeks of taking six capsules per day. The bleeding and diarrhea were noticeably less severe. I had a nearly normal, firm stool and the bleeding had stopped within one month. After two months, I had two normal bowel movements per day. I can eat anything I want again. I feel absolutely great!

"The other interesting thing is that I have tried three different brands of colostrum," Lawrence says. "Two of them did nothing. Only when I took this 'first-milking' colostrum did the symptoms subside and stay in check."

Viruses

Viruses are extremely tiny—much smaller than bacteria. They invade individual cells and turn them into tiny factories to make more viruses. The pharmaceutical community has developed antibiotic after antibiotic to target an ever-growing group of bacterial pathogens, yet few medicines today work on viral infections. Health-care practitioners have little ammunition when it comes to viruses.

Viral diseases include colds and flu, chicken pox, hepatitis, measles, herpes, viral pneumonia, shingles, Epstein Barr virus, respiratory syncytial virus (RSV), AIDS, and numerous others. There are also a host of intestinal viruses that cause diarrhea and other life-threatening symptoms. Viruses cause serious health difficulties each year.

Colostrum also aids our fight against viruses. In the last few years, colostrum and a number of its individual components have been seriously studied for their effects against a variety of viral diseases. As with the bacterial pathogens, colostrum's ability to help with viral infections is more likely due to immune support and the combination of substances than to any specific antibody reaction.

Colostrum's anti-viral properties include:

- Lactoferrin, an iron binding protein with antiviral, antibacterial, and anti-inflammatory properties. It is currently being studied for its effects against the HIV virus, herpes, and even cancer.

- Cytokines, which regulate the intensity of the immune response. They are known to boost the production of antibodies important in fighting viral infections.

- Leukocytes, the white blood cells that engulf invading organisms, including viruses.

So far, vaccinations have been our only defense against the viral population. Perhaps this is the reason why numerous studies have focused on creating specific antibodies in colostrum by injecting a virus into a pregnant cow and then collecting the resulting colostrum. The resulting colostrum can be made to contain specific antibodies for viral organisms such as rotavirus. This colostrum, called hyper immune colostrum, has been shown to be very effective in eradicating viral pathogens. Someday, we may all be able to choose our vaccinations from hyper immune colostrum.

Certainly, colostrum provides components that boost the immune response and build up a weakened immune system. Sometimes colostrum provides enough of an immune boost for people to turn the corner and begin to win the war against viral pathogens. In other cases, the extra energy is enough to relieve symptoms even while the virus is still present.

FYI: Colostrum vs. AIDS

The best example of immunodeficiency is Acquired Immune Deficiency Syndrome, or AIDS. Individuals with AIDS have such a suppressed immune response that a cold or flu can be devastating. What often happens with AIDS patients is that they are left vulnerable to viral and bacterial infections that settle in the bowel, thereby causing diarrhea. A 1992 study with immune-deficient patients experiencing chronic diarrhea due to viral infections showed that 72 percent experienced stool normalization after 10 days of treatment with concentrated bovine colostral immunoglobulins. Other studies have shown similar results. For persons suffering from immune suppression and immunodeficient patients, colostrum can be very helpful, perhaps even lifesaving.

CLINICAL CASE REPORT: Jill S.

Three years ago, Jill S. of North Altamonte Springs, Florida, was diagnosed with active Epstein Barr virus. "I was tired and achy all the time," she recalls. "I had swollen glands and a constant sore throat. Although I was never actually bedridden, the continual fatigue was trying.

"When I began taking first-milking colostrum, I initially felt very sick. Then I got my strength back, the aches and pains subsided and the perpetual sore throat went away. I actually quit taking the colostrum to prove to myself that there was a difference. Sure enough, in about five days the aches and pains began again and I felt that familiar sore throat coming back. Within a couple of days after taking colostrum again, the symptoms disappeared."

Fungi

Fungi are everywhere. These single-celled organisms can be found in the air, water, and soil. They are normal inhabitants of the skin, gastrointestinal and genitourinary tracts. They can be very helpful in digestion, in the synthesis of vitamins, and in the prevention of infections. They become a problem only when they get out of balance with other intestinal flora.

Candida is a fungus that can overgrow and destroy the balance of microbes in the gastrointestinal tract. When it is maintained in a normal ratio, Candida represents about 1 in every 100,000 beneficial microbes. Candida only becomes a problem when the balance of normal flora is disrupted. Once out of control, it shifts from an overgrowth into a fungal form and grows roots that reach into the intestinal lining, making it very difficult to treat. An overgrowth further irritates the intestinal lining and weakens the whole immune system.

Candida is in epidemic proportions in our society today due to the long-term use of antibiotics and the poor quality of food we consume. Symptoms of Candida can vary widely, but include vaginal and mouth eruptions, skin irritations such as eczema and dermatitis, food sensitivities, nutritional deficiency due to malabsorption, irregular bowel movements, fatigue, headaches, and bloating.

Although studies elaborate on the ability of colostral components to inhibit the growth of Candida, it is probably due to an indirect action rather than an actual effect on the Candida itself. Colostrum works to heal the lining of the intestinal tract, sealing abnormal holes that cause a whole cascade of events known as "leaky gut syndrome." When a leaky gut is healed, it becomes much less susceptible to Candida overgrowth and to a whole compliment of difficulties that might result.

However, once Candida has become rooted in the lining of the intestinal tract, it is very difficult to control. Use of colostrum can lessen the symptoms and help heal the lining of the intestines, but since Candida is such a huge problem and since so many individuals have it in fungal form, modifications in diet, along with the use of other supplements, are usually necessary to control the problem.

Parasites

Everything that we once took for granted is changing—especially when it comes to our health and safety. We may have once thought that here in America, our exposure to parasites and mycoplasmas (a type of parasite) is highly limited. But this just isn't so. Many health conditions for which there seem to be no good answers remain unsolved only because the patient and doctor failed to appreciate the high frequency of parasitical or mycoplasma infection, even among persons living in the United States.

In tests performed in clinics from New York to Arizona and by the Centers for Disease Control and Prevention, it is apparent that the U.S. has one of the highest rates of parasitic infestations in the world. As a matter of fact, U.S. rates are five times higher than Mexico in five pathogenic parasites. It is dangerous and foolish to think that parasites are a third world problem!

Take the West Nile virus, which causes encephalitis, an inflammation of the brain. West Nile virus was once commonly found only in Africa, West Asia, and the Middle East, but in 1999, its presence was documented in the United States.

Signs posted in wilderness areas often warn about *Giardia* in streams. Commonly found in wild animals such as the beaver, this graceful, flagellated organism may infect unwary hikers. However, giardiasis can also be contracted via contaminated foods. There is some evidence that a heavy infection of attached *Giardia* physically blocks the important transport of nutrients across the epithelium, the thin layer of tissue covering organs, glands and other structures in the body.

Entamoeba histolytica, another water-borne pathogen, can cause diarrhea or a more serious invasive liver abscess. When in contact with human cells, these amoebas cause a rapid influx of calcium into the cells, disrupting functions and causing the cells to die. The amoeba may eat the dead cell or just absorb nutrients released from the cell.

Parasites are much more common than we have been willing to admit, and they have been shown to be involved with many kinds of disease. Miron G. Shultz, M.D., director of the Parasitic Diseases Division of the U.S. Centers for Disease Control and Prevention, notes that "protozoa and helminths (worms) are causing many diseases that baffle doctors." For example, mycoplasma, an insidious type of parasite that is very difficult to eliminate, has been linked with Gulf War Syndrome and a number of other health problems whose treatment has been elusive.

According to University of Texas researchers Joel B. Baseman and Joseph G. Tully: "Recently, mycoplasmas have been linked as a cofactor to AIDS pathogenesis and to malignant transformation, chromosomal aberrations, the Gulf War Syndrome, and other unexplained and complex illnesses including chronic fatigue syndrome, Crohn's disease, and various arthritides...they are evolutionarily advanced, and their elite status as 'next generation' bacterial pathogens necessitates new paradigms in fully understanding their disease potential."

Parasites thrive in a body with a compromised immune system where the intestinal flora is out of balance. Parasites compete with us for nutrients and secrete toxic waste products that add to the burden of the immune system.

Colostrum can help with both of these, strengthening the immune system and contributing to the health of the intestinal tract. So although colostrum may not fight parasites directly, it can definitely influence the internal terrain of the gastrointestinal tract and aid in preventing parasitic infections.

Common intestinal symptoms that many experience as a result of parasites include bloating, diarrhea, flatulence, cramps, and constipation. Parasites can be symptomatic of irritable bowel syndrome, colitis, and leaky gut. Often, clients diagnosed with chronic fatigue, allergies, memory loss, skin disorders, and muscle pain are experiencing the results of parasites and never realize it!

Identifying parasite infection is providing relief for many with so-called "mysterious" illnesses. According to Garth Nicolson, Ph.D. and Nancy Nicolson, Ph.D. at the Institute for Molecular Medicine in Huntington Beach, Calif., thousands of Gulf War soldiers are finally being helped now that mycoplasma infections have been identified and eliminated from their bodies.

And, identifying the presence of parasitical and mycoplasma infections in patients with chronic fatigue immune deficiency syndrome (CFIDS), fibromyalgia, and rheumatoid arthritis enables health care professionals to rule out other causes of illness. At the Life Sources Clinic in Fair Oaks, Calif., where health professionals work with live blood microscopy, Dr. Hugh Smith notes, "We've definitively linked parasites and mycoplasmas with multiple sclerosis, lupus and other autoimmune disorders, as well as irritable bowel syndrome and digestive disorders."

Other experts have observed mycoplasma-damaged red blood cells in a consistently growing percentage of patients. In these cases, the treatment process is simple and direct–eliminate the mycoplasma and reverse the damage done. While this may seem simplistic, keep this caveat in mind; one may generally assume as a rule of thumb that reversal of disease requires one month for every year of suffering.

CLINICAL CASE REPORT: Amy D.

Several months ago, Amy D. of Tucson, Arizona, began experiencing a number of symptoms. "Initially, I noticed an emptiness after meals, then bloating and gas. Later, I began to have a tightness under my breastbone, a lump in my throat and often a shortness of breath. Skin problems also developed. These were so unusual for me that I decided to go to a natural doctor.

"I visited an iridologist, who told me I had parasites. He gave me an herbal detox and first-milking colostrum, which I took for a month. When I returned a month later, feeling much better, he told me there was no longer evidence of the parasitic infection. I feel like colostrum played a big role in the elimination of these parasites, and I plan to continue taking it."

Chapter 6

Colostrum and Autoimmune Diseases

What happens when the immune system fails to distinguish "self" from "other"? What happens when the immune system attacks its own host—you?

Two words: autoimmune disease, which appears to be on the rise in industrialized nations.

You may not know them as autoimmune conditions, but some of the more common autoimmune diseases include: lupus, rheumatoid arthritis, multiple sclerosis, Addison's disease, childhood asthma, fibromyalgia, chronic fatigue syndrome, scleroderma, thyroiditis, vasculitis, Crohn's disease, colitis, Raynaud's disease, and others. These conditions result when ongoing allergic reactions trigger a hyper-immune response, resulting in an attack on the body itself.

These types of diseases have been somewhat of a mystery to healthcare professionals; most recommended treatments simply provide minor relief of pain and other symptoms. The real answer lies in enhancing the body's healing response—the return to dynamic homeostasis, or balance of the immune system.

As discussed in Chapter 3, the PRP found in colostrum, with its ability to regulate overactive immune response, can be indispensable to persons with autoimmune disease. Other factors contained in colostrum repeatedly contribute to the healing of the intestinal lining; in some cases of autoimmune disease we find that triggering agents filter from the "leaky" gut into the bloodstream.

This is why individuals with autoimmune diseases usually respond so well to colostrum—it helps to repair the gut that may be leaking antigens into the bloodstream that trigger an autoimmune response.

Reverse Healing

People with autoimmune diseases who start using colostrum almost always experience a healing crisis—a process known as "reverse healing." This means that at the beginning of the body's healing response, they experience more severe symptoms for a short period of time. Often, they re-experience the symptoms of their condition as it developed over the years—only this time in reverse order. As healing takes place, they generally have a greater sense of well-being, and their symptoms lessen.

"One patient had three autoimmune conditions: chronic fatigue, fibromyalgia, and lupus," notes naturopathic doctor Thomas Stone. "She wanted to be able to make a full-time commitment to her work, but her health would not allow it. When I told her about my program, which includes dietary changes and colostrum, she indicated her desire to move at a pace that would allow her to get through the healing crisis as quickly as possible.

"When she began, she became bedridden for about one week. However, when she got her energy back, she told me she couldn't remember feeling as good. The majority of her symptoms were gone within one month. I don't usually recommend that my patients move that quickly, but this particular woman had reasons for needing to proceed in the way that she did.

"If people are willing to make the changes in lifestyle, and to take colostrum faithfully, most people with autoimmune diseases are pleasantly surprised—especially when they have been given little hope of relief from other courses of action."

Let's take a look at how first-milking colostrum can help other specific autoimmune conditions.

Systemic Lupus Erythematosus (SLE or Lupus)

Systemic lupus erythematosus is a chronic inflammatory disease in which the body's immune system fails to serve its normal protective functions. Instead, it forms antibodies that attack healthy tissues and organs. For many people, lupus is a mild disease; for others, it may cause serious and even life-threatening problems. If left untreated, lupus can be fatal.

Lupus, like many autoimmune disorders, may be a result of infection by stealth pathogens (e.g., mycoplasmas) that escape initial immune detection. Lupus most often strikes young women between the ages of 20 to 40. The condition is characterized by severe fatigue and a butterfly rash across the face. Debilitating pain and swelling often occur in the hands, wrists, elbows, knees, ankles, or feet. There may also be morning stiffness in the joints, a pale or blue tinge to the fingers when exposed to cold, and possibly hair loss.

Lupus is one of the most complex and vicious autoimmune diseases and can attack almost any cell in the body. It is much more prevalent in females than males and is more common in Asians and African Americans than Caucasians. The disease is not restricted to humans and occurs in other species, including dogs and rodents. Once diagnosed, the disease is usually controlled based upon symptoms, most frequently using corticosteroids. However, it can suddenly fulminate and frequently is terminal. Patients suffer from periodic outbursts of pain associated with organ inflammation and are frequently lethargic with low energy due to an associated hemolytic anemia. Lupus may also cause diseases of the internal organs, including the heart, brain, lungs, and kidneys, as well as bleeding, anemia, and chronic infections. It is not unusual for lupus patients to require kidney transplants.

With proper treatment, lupus can be controlled, and sufferers can expect normal life expectancy. However, patients with lupus are frequently placed on high dose cortisone for long periods of time.

Routine use of high quality colostrum can offer significant help.

The IGF-I and 87 proteins in the IGF super family assist in the regeneration and repair of damaged cells. The IGF-I provided by colostrum results in improved metabolism of glucose to glycogen,

FYI: Rheumatoid Arthritis & Leaky Gut

Some experts believe that rheumatoid arthritis can be caused by allergens, especially those in the diet, combined with a permeable intestinal wall (leaky gut wall syndrome) that allows large undigested food particles to pass through. They believe that this initiates the immune response that eventually leads to the disabling and painful inflammation associated with rheumatoid arthritis.

James Braly, M.D., medical director of Immuno Laboratories, Inc., of Fort Lauderdale, Florida, notes: "Five to 10 years ago, it would have been heresy to state that allergens could induce arthritis and that by the elimination of those allergens, the arthritis would go into remission. Now it's accepted among most rheumatologists and allergists that some people do have allergy-induced arthritis. A primary cause of most rheumatoid arthritis appears to be delayed food allergy, and the often related problem of abnormal permeability of the intestinal wall [leaky gut syndrome]."

According to this theory, partially digested food particles pass through the intestinal wall into the bloodstream. These unintentional "invaders" are then deposited in the body's joints and other tissues where they can cause an inflammatory response as the body's immune system mobilizes to disarm them.

Less known is that bacterial infections may also be at the root of some cases of rheumatoid arthritis. Other microbial invaders, including protozoa, yeast, and fungus, can also cause or aggravate arthritis. Some medical agents like diuretics may trigger arthritis. Finally, some people (albeit a small percentage), may simply inherit their condition.

It is highly likely that if you routinely supplement your diet with colostrum, some of the symptoms that you are experiencing will be relieved. In addition, colostrum can potentially help with the damaging side effects of commonly used over-the-counter drugs.

For example, the nonsteroidal anti-inflammatory drugs (e.g., NSAIDs such as aspirin and ibuprofen) that people take can be highly inflammatory to the lining of the gastrointestinal tract. In some cases, these NSAIDs will trigger a condition known as leaky gut where the spaces between the epithelial cells lining the intestinal wall widen. This can cause extreme gastrointestinal distress and, in some cases, makes the individual more susceptible to infections in the intestines. Routine use of a high quality colostrum product has been shown to significantly relieve this condition.

Since certain aspects of this disease are autoimmune, this represents an immune system that is out of control, and the best way to put things back into place naturally is via colostrum. The growth factors in colostrum help restore the thymus, considered the seat of the immune system, to normal function. In addition, colostrum's proline-rich polypeptide helps to keep the immune system under control.

yielding more energy and diminishing lethargy. IGF-I also improves the metabolism of amino acids to proteins, helping in cell repair and replacement of damaged proteins.

Susan R. of Toluca Lake, Calif., suffered from systemic lupus for five years with symptoms that allowed her to continue to work but, nevertheless, left her with a feeling of complete exhaustion.

"The biggest difficulty was the exhaustion," Susan says. "By the time Friday afternoon came around, I was so exhausted that all I could do was fall into bed at the end of the day. I usually spent all day Saturday resting—building up enough energy to do the laundry, clean up the apartment and get ready to do it all over again the next week."

Her sister told her about colostrum, having read a book about its use by patients with lupus and other autoimmune disorders. Susan began taking three capsules, two times per day. What do I have to lose? she thought to herself.

"The following Friday, I stopped off on the way home from work and bought new pots for my houseplants. I went home and repotted all my plants, vacuumed my apartment and made a nice dinner for myself. At 9 p.m., I was ready to mop the kitchen floor when I suddenly realized what I had done. It was Friday night, and I was full of energy. I called my sister in utter amazement! That was six months ago, but it was the beginning of a whole new pattern in my life."

Since then, Susan has continued to see benefits from taking colostrum. She's lost weight, her legs don't burn when she walks, and she has emerged from what patients commonly call her "lupus fog." "My boss at work even asked me what I was doing because I am so much more on top of things," she says.

Susan found a natural agent that helped to normalize her immune function. Perhaps the immune factors in colostrum were able to help Susan finally quell this infection.

Rheumatoid Arthritis

Rheumatoid arthritis is a chronic disease of the joints characterized by periods of active inflammation. The joints may become just a little stiff at first, but a few weeks later, they become much stiffer and more swollen. The stiffness and swelling may start in the small joints like the fingers and wrists, but progress to larger joints and afflict both the joints and bodily organs. About one-third of rheumatoid arthritis patients get luckier than most, with only a single joint area or two being affected. Even so, this is a total disease, affecting the body inside and out.

Between 8 and 10 million Americans have rheumatoid arthritis. Rheumatoid arthritis is most likely to strike women aged 36 to 50, according to the National Rheumatism Foundation. The next major target is men 45 to 60. Occasionally, even children and teenagers suffer various forms of rheumatoid arthritis.

Ordinarily, the immune system repels threats to health from bacteria, viruses, and chemical toxins, as well as diseased, damaged cells. Thankfully, our immune system's powerful yet complex army of defenders—its B cells, T cells, antibodies, and macrophages (debris eaters)—generally eat up, digest, and otherwise disarm real threats to our health.

In rheumatoid arthritis, however, the immune system is out of control and it turns against the body. Although medical science is unsure of the exact cause of rheumatoid arthritis, we do know that for some reason the body's immune system begins to form antibodies that cause a chronic inflammation of the joints.

In normal individuals, the B cells produce antibodies that attack and defuse foreign substances (i.e., viruses and toxins) in the body. In people with rheumatoid arthritis, however, these antibodies and foreign matter form large immune complexes so misshapen and foreign to the body itself that they themselves are attacked by the immune system, resulting in inflammation and joint destruction. As these attacks continue to occur, the bones and joint tissues are weakened and eventually destroyed, destroying the integrity of the joint, including the cartilage that provides a cushioning effect. This battle within the immune system is likely to spread throughout the body, damaging and killing off the red blood cells. This leads to symptoms like weakness, fatigue, and swelling.

The formation of these new antibodies may be heightened due to a variety of influences on a patient's health. One's genes, for example, may make one vulnerable to foreign toxins and pathogens such as food allergies and biological pathogens such as bacteria and viruses, which can initiate an immune firestorm. However, lifestyle and diet can also contribute to the firestorm, as can allergies.

People like Jackie T. of Avon Park, Flor., have seen colostrum greatly improve their arthritis problems. "I used to have arthritis so badly that I couldn't close my hands completely," says Jackie. "My knuckles were badly swollen and my fingers were so misshapen and stiff that I couldn't lay my hands flat on a table. I began taking four capsules of colostrum a day, and within two months, I could make a fist again. With that encouragement, I increased my dosage to 10 capsules a day and began to notice that the swelling in my knuckles was slowly going down.

"Today, one year later, I can stretch my hand out flat on the table, and the size of my knuckles is at least a half inch less than it used to be," Jackie says happily. "Besides that, my complexion is better and I just plain feel healthier."

Larry H. of Chicago, Ill., has also seen great benefits from taking colostrum. After suffering from rheumatoid arthritis for 25 years and more recently being diagnosed with fibromyalgia, Larry was desperate for help.

"I have experienced more than my share of aches and pains," Larry says. "But even more debilitating than the pain and stiffness was the lack of energy. For about two years, if I wanted to do anything, I almost had to build up the energy for several days beforehand and then rest for an equal amount of time afterward— just to be able to do simple things like go shopping.

"All that has changed. Within about a week after I began taking colostrum, I woke up one morning and I actually felt human. Ever since then, I have been able to do the things I used to do. My whole outlook on life has changed. I am no longer depressed. I have the energy that I did when I was 30 years old. I frequently forget to take that second arthritis pill in the afternoon and it hasn't seemed to matter. The longer I take colostrum, the better it gets."

Multiple Sclerosis

Multiple Sclerosis (MS) is a tragic disease. It strikes relatively young persons and has no known cure. More than one million individuals worldwide suffer from MS.

The disease is seen much more frequently in cold, damp regions than in the warmer countries. For example, in Germany alone, some 100,000 individuals suffer from MS. Independent of these climactic zones, however, specific population groups are afflicted more frequently with this disease. MS occurs about twice as frequently among women as in men, and it usually begins between the ages of 15 and 40.

MS is the third highest cause of severe disability in patients in the United States between the ages of 15 and 50, reports Reuven Sandyk, M.D., in the *Journal of Alternative and Complementary Medicine.*

"The cause of the disease and its pathogenesis remain unknown," states Sandyk. "The last 20 years have seen only meager advances in the development of effective treatments for the disease. No specific treatment modality can cure the disease or alter its long-term course and eventual outcome. Moreover, there have been no agents that restore . . . neuronal functions."

There are a variety of therapies currently used for MS: numerous drug therapies, steroids, cortisones, Beta-interferon, synthetic protein injection (Copolymer-1), immunosuppressants (cyclophosphamide, azathioprine, and cyclosporine), and even lymphoid irradiation. However, many of the therapies have numerous side effects and/or unknown long-term effects.

Previous virological and immunological studies have suggested that multiple sclerosis is an autoimmune disease triggered by a virus infection. Dr. Y. Ohara of the Department of Microbiology, Kanazawa Medical University, Ishikawa, Japan, suggests that patients with MS are exposed to some infectious agent or combination of agents before puberty. The presence of virus-induced demyelination in animal models (demyelination is the major underlying factor responsible for the symptoms of MS and involves the destructive removal of myelin, an insulating and protective fatty protein which sheaths nerve cells) indicates that demyelination can occur following the trigger of a virus infection.

One such viral agent is the measles virus, which may be a causative agent of the demyelination observed in MS. Research has shown that MS patients have far higher levels of antibodies against the disease than others, indicating that the immune system of these people is constantly reacting to such an infection. (However, it has not been determined whether it originates from a natural infection or is the result of a measles vaccine.) While the measles virus may not always be involved, it certainly appears to be a causative factor or contributor to disease in a significant number of MS patients. Another is the Epstein-Barr virus, which is linked with mononucleosis.

Because of this, a specially developed type of hyper immune colostrum could hold one of the keys to healing MS patients. When cows are exposed to the measles virus, they produce a type of colostrum that is rich in measles-specific antibodies. These antibodies confer a passive immunity to the person who consumes the bovine colostrum. (The cows eventually get over their case of measles.) With this added immunity, the MS patient's immune system can decimate the measles virus, initiating the healing process.

This theory was put to the test in a study published in 1984, when a specially produced colostrum was orally administered every morning to 15 patients with MS at a daily dosage of 100 milliliters for 30 days. A measles-negative antibody control colostrum was orally administered to 5 patients. Among seven high-symptom patients, five recipients improved and two remained unchanged. Among eight low-symptom patients, five patients improved and three remained unchanged. Among those receiving the placebo, two patients remained unchanged and three worsened. No side effects were observed in colostrum recipients.

The growth factors in colostrum are also highly beneficial for MS sufferers. Insulin-like growth factor-I, platelet-derived growth factor (PDGF), fibroblast growth factor (FGF), and ciliary neurotrophic factor (CNTF) are multifunctional growth factors that promote the proliferation, differentiation, and survival of cells. Since myelin breakdown is often severe in MS, the possibility of growth factor use in the treatment of MS has been considered. Recently, IGF-I treatment has been shown to reduce lesion severity and promote myelin regeneration in experimental autoimmune encephalomyelitis (EAE), an animal model of MS.

Many health experts now believe that autoimmune conditions stem from viral or bacterial infections. Most recently, researchers have linked multiple sclerosis to the virus that causes mononucleosis. We have strong reason to believe that if every child were given additional colostrum, our incidence of autoimmune disease would decrease significantly.

Crohn's Disease

Crohn's disease causes inflammation in the small intestine, and can also affect any part of the digestive tract from the mouth to the anus.

The inflammation can cause pain and can make the intestines empty frequently, resulting in diarrhea.

It has long been known that the development of Crohn's disease somehow involves infection with *Mycobacterium paratuberculosis*, a relative of the bacterium that causes tuberculosis. Researchers originally believed that it was the primary cause of the disease, but now recognize that there are autoimmune manifestations associated with the disease.

Routine utilization of very high quality bovine colostrum can be very advantageous to people with Crohn's. IGF-I helps to regulate the metabolic pathway by which the body converts glucose (sugar) to glycogen (glycogen is stored in the muscles and the liver and is the main source of energy when the muscles are exercised). Another major function of IGF-I and the "superfamily" is regulating how cells use amino acids to build proteins. Having sufficient IGF-I available is extremely important in metabolically compromised individuals and is essential to reversing the wasting aspects of the disease.

Another function of the IGF superfamily is the repair of damaged cells. Most of the proteins in the superfamily are present in almost every cell in the body, but require activation and direction by the attachment of IGF-I to specific sites on a cell's surface. Again, having sufficient IGF-I available is critical for cell repair.

Colostrum also contains a number of gut protective factors that can act in concert to control infections. Some of the most important ones are:

- The IgA immunoglobulins directed against various bacteria and viruses like E. coli, Staph. aureus, and others that can attack the gut and, more particularly, weakened tissue. IgA will not only attach itself to a microorganism, but can also attach itself to tissue and immobilize the invading agent, letting other factors act to destroy it.

- Lactoferrin and transferrin are iron-binding proteins. Certain bacteria and viruses that invade the gut require iron to reproduce. When this substance is withheld, they die.

- Lysozyme and lactoperoxidase are powerful enzymes that can attach to bacteria and eat holes through their outer wall.

With such an abundance of benefits for the body's immune system, colostrum's potential for helping autoimmune sufferers holds great promise.

FYI: Importance of Quality Colostrum for Autoimmune Conditions

When using colostrum for autoimmune disorders, it's of extreme importance to ensure that a substantial portion of these biologically active substances gets through the stomach and into the intestines where they are needed. Accomplishing this is simple: use a complete first-milking colostrum that contains all of the fat and casein. The human stomach contains an enzyme, rennin, that is also found in bovines and other species. Rennin acts on the fat and casein in dairy products to form a soft cheese-like curd that protects the biologically active substances against the enzymes and acid environment of the stomach, allowing the substances to either pass through within the curd as it disintegrates and/or to be absorbed into the circulation.

Chapter 7

Colostrum, Blood Sugar Levels and Insulin

> "I was so depressed and sick for almost two years with diabetes, fibromyalgia, osteoporosis and osteoarthritis, that I didn't really care anymore. I was too sick to support myself, and I didn't know how I would get through each day.
>
> "When I began taking colostrum, the first thing I noticed was that my appetite changed. With diabetes, you can eat a big meal and still feel hungry. After several weeks on the colostrum, I didn't feel hungry anymore. I noticed that my energy was increasing and that I wasn't as depressed.
>
> "Then I noticed that my blood sugar levels were changing. With careful monitoring (two to four times a day), I have been able to lower my insulin from 96 units/day to 10 units/day during the last 9 months. I used to take lots of pain medication, now I take none—a good warm bath is all I need to help with occasional pain from overwork. I am working again and supporting myself after two years of not being able to. I have also lost weight—it almost rolled off me as the severe swelling in my whole body disappeared. All this didn't happen at once, so I would encourage people to have patience."
>
> - Pat B., Ontario, Canada

The American Diabetes Association has estimated that one in every 14 people in the United States either has or will have diabetes during their lifetime.

Diabetes is generally divided into two categories. Type 2 diabetes often does not require insulin, although it can develop to the point where insulin is required. Type 1 diabetes is often referred to as juvenile onset diabetes and can progress rapidly. Frequently, it develops as an autoimmune disease, where antibodies attack the insulin-producing cells of the pancreas.

One early treatment for this form of diabetes is the use of immunosuppressive drugs, which may cause other complications. As a viable alternative, colostrum contains proline-rich polypeptide (PRP), which has been shown to balance the overactive immune response associated with autoimmune diseases. Rather than suppressing the immune system with drugs, colostrum can balance overactive immune responses to reduce the attack on pancreatic cells.

Diabetes requires careful dietary and exercise programs. Even though type 2 is a milder form, it is not without secondary complications including heart disease, kidney disease, atherosclerosis, vision problems, and circulatory problems. Those with diabetes, regardless of the type, are five times more likely to develop cardiovascular disease than those without diabetes. Incidentally, diabetes is sometimes diagnosed for the first time following a heart attack. That's why it's good to know that colostrum can help to regrow heart tissue and supporting blood vessels, and reduce the bacteria associated with arterial plaque.

Colostrum has also been shown to balance blood sugar levels. This is due, at least in part, to the growth factor IGF-I. A 1990 edition of *Diabetes* suggested that colostrum supplementation would be a very beneficial treatment for diabetes, based on the fact that IGF-I can stimulate glucose utilization. (Researchers found that IGF-I levels were lower in diabetic patients than in healthy individuals. After administering IGF-I to patients, doctors noticed a two-fold increase in glucose transport to the muscles, potentially treating hyperglycemia and the dependence on insulin.)

Be careful though to select a first-milking colostrum, says a health expert. "As a naturopathic physician, I was using colostrum 20 years ago. Back then, I could get it from organic farmers in the

Midwest, and I used it in liquid form. However, when I moved my practice, I was no longer able to obtain it from the local farmers, so I investigated numerous forms of dried colostrum on the market. None of them even came close to the track record I had established with true colostrum, so I eliminated it from my practice for a number of years.

"Finally, several years ago, I discovered [commercially available true first-milking colostrum]. Just tasting and feeling it, I knew I had found the real thing. And sure enough, when I gave this to my patients, they experienced the benefits I knew they could. Once again, colostrum has become an integral part of my practice.

"For diabetic patients, colostrum is unbeatable. Within months, every one of my patients have either greatly reduced their levels of insulin or have eliminated it altogether. That's quite a track record, but it's true. Of course, they are also drinking plenty of good water, exercising, and eating an enhanced diet of 'live, whole foods,' but it is the colostrum which makes the program work. Given enough time, colostrum can completely eliminate the need for insulin. It balances the pancreas just like it does the thymus so that blood sugar levels are able to normalize.

"I have also used colostrum with a product called Hydroxygen Plus for the resolution of diabetic ulcers on legs and feet. As a poultice, it heals ulcers untreatable by conventional methods. Most ulcers of this nature will heal within a matter of weeks. For the diabetic, colostrum is a Godsend—literally!"

Please note that, especially with insulin-dependant patients, it is very important to consult a health care practitioner before taking colostrum and/or making changes in medication.

Chapter 8

Colostrum for Athletes and Staying in Shape

Colostrum benefits the athlete in so many ways that it is rapidly gaining in popularity—especially amongst those who prefer to stay with natural substances. Athletes and those who exercise or work out regularly share a number of common denominators that make them prime candidates for colostrum. Not only does it help build lean muscle tissue, colostrum also slows protein breakdown and speeds protein synthesis. In fact, many body builders say that colostrum is the most effective muscle-building agent they have ever used!

The 1988 and 1992 Jamaican Olympic silver medalist Winthrop Graham discovered first-milking colostrum after suffering a knee injury in the 1996 Olympics. "It was a rather serious injury and doctors wanted to perform surgery, but I opted for a rehabilitation program," says Graham, a hurdlist.

Two years passed, but he was still having trouble recovering after running the hurdles. His knee would become stiff and prevent him from training consistently. However, within two months after he began taking first-milking colostrum, he says, "I could run the hurdles with no stiffness at all," he says. "That was amazing to me, and I became a believer."

For bodybuilder Jeff S., first-milking colostrum helped him to realize his dreams. "I always wanted to be a bodybuilder, so I tried everything natural to gain weight and build muscle. Nothing had any significant effect until I found colostrum," Jeff says.

He began taking a half-teaspoon twice a day, and immediately noticed how much better he felt. He increased his workouts to six hours per day, seven days a week. He lost 25 pounds, adding lean muscle to become one "ripped" dude.

"People stop me on the street and say, 'I don't mean to embarrass you but you have the most incredible body.' No one ever said that kind of thing to me before. My friends who knew me can't believe I've lost weight because they can see I'm bigger. It's so amazing!"

These days, Jeff uses two to three heaping teaspoons of colostrum powder four times per day and is devoted full-time to bodybuilding.

"Tree surgeon" David K. maintains demanding weight training sessions in order to stay fit. "I have tried a number of things, including a homeopathic form of human growth hormone, but I have never been able to really gain weight," he says. "My weight stayed relatively constant for 30 years—between 190 and 200 pounds—until I started taking colostrum. After three months, I weighed 220 with no increase in body fat."

Colostrum for Tissue Repair and Recovery

Each time we exercise strenuously, we cause tiny tears in muscle tissue. The growth factors in colostrum help to quickly repair this damage, strengthening muscles. The regenerative effects of colostrum extend to nearly all structural cells of the body; in fact, IGF-I is the best known compound for synthesis and repair of cartilage. Other compounds known as transforming growth factors A and B are known for their ability to enhance healing and for taking part in the synthesis and repair of both RNA and DNA.

Most athletes using colostrum report quicker recovery without the same level of fatigue. For example, several years ago, the Finnish Olympic ski team participated in a study involving colostrum. Members of the team who took colostrum showed significantly reduced muscle-cell damage on the fourth day following seven days of acute exercise. They also reported being less fatigued.

For athletes interested in enhanced physical performance, the scientific evidence supporting use of colostrum is noteworthy. Its high content of bioactive growth factors like IGF-I and hGH is generating interest among sports doctors. Growth factors are made up of short protein chains called polypeptides that play key regulatory roles in cell growth, replication, and differentiation. Growth factors support complex feedback loops between the immune, nervous, and hormonal systems that maintain healthy homeostasis under normal circumstances.

Colostrum Builds Lean Muscle

One of the difficulties with achieving muscular development lies not just in building muscle, but also in preventing muscle breakdown. Paradoxically, the exercise that is required to build muscle can also be the very thing that causes muscle breakdown.

A true first-milking colostrum addresses both ends of this dilemma. It contains a whole complex of compounds that work to build lean muscle mass and burn fat rather than muscle. Research has shown that during exercise, IGF-I is the signal that triggers muscle cell proliferation, working hand in hand with human growth hormone (hGH) and other components for the building of lean muscle mass. Most athletes are extremely impressed with colostrum's ability to enhance muscle development.

The same growth factors that work to build lean muscle also play a pivotal role in preventing muscle breakdown during exercise. During heavy workouts and in times of hunger, the body tends to burn protein instead of fat. Since IGF-I governs the synthesis of protein from amino acids, having an abundance of this factor in the system means that muscle need not be burned for fuel during heavy workouts; rather, more fat is utilized.

Colostrum Boosts Stamina

Athletes require strength and stamina to compete. Anything that will enhance endurance and maximize fuel is certainly an asset. The growth factors contained in colostrum shift fuel utilization from carbohydrate to fat, actually preventing the body from burning glucose for energy.

Colostrum Supports Athletic Immune System

Because intense athletic endeavors actually depress the immune system immediately following a period of activity, athletes such as marathoners and bodybuilders are prone to infections and other illnesses. Factors contained in colostrum can make a remarkable difference in preventing illness for athletes. Both the growth factors and immune factors found in colostrum continually work to strengthen the immune system so that vulnerability after exercise is less of an issue. The growth hormones in colostrum, particularly hGH, help the body produce antibodies, T-cells, and other white blood cells; together with IGF-I, hGH has been used quite successfully to fight off infection. This is why athletes who take colostrum experience shorter recovery times, indicating less "down time" for the immune system.

Roger J. of Santa Monica, Calif. used colostrum to help with his chronic fatigue and can now enjoy the vigorous exercise his condition forced him to reduce. "I have had chronic fatigue for seven years. Besides the lack of energy, I also gradually lost the strength and stamina to exercise the way I had always done. Now, with colostrum, I am running two to four miles, five days a week and also aggressively working out five days a week—without inflammation or other symptoms."

Colostrum Aids Nutrient Uptake

Nutrition is of paramount importance to athletes. Making sure the body has sufficient nutrients for strenuous exercise and the building blocks for repair is essential.

That's why the support that colostrum offers the entire digestive system is important. Colostrum heals the lining of the digestive tract where nutrient absorption takes place. Not only does this enhance nutrient uptake, it also prevents invading organisms from attaching to the intestinal lining and causing infection. This also explains the boost in energy that many people feel when they take colostrum.

Better Sports Performance with Colostrum: Studies

Exercise and training results in muscle damage which, in turn, reduces performance during subsequent exercise. Colostrum seems to counteract this negative effect. Let's look at some of the research on colostrum and physical fitness.

Study #1: Increases in IGF-I. In a study from the Department of Biology of Physical Activity, University of Jyväskylä, Finland, researchers examined the effects of bovine colostrum supplementation on serum IGF-I concentrations in the bodies of athletes during a strength and speed training period. Nine male sprinters and jumpers underwent three randomized experimental training treatments of eight days separated by 13 days. One group consumed 125 milliliters of colostrum, while a placebo group was given normal milk whey.

Post-training increases were noticed for serum IGF-I levels in the colostrum group as compared with the placebo group. "It appears that a bovine colostrum supplement . . . may increase serum IGF-I concentration in athletes during strength and speed training," noted the researchers.

Study #2: Better Performance & Lower Serum Creatine Kinase. At the Center for Research in Education and Sports Science at the University of South Australia, a double-blind, placebo controlled study was carried out to determine the effect of supplementation with a commercial bovine colostrum product on plasma IGF-I concentrations and endurance running performance.

In the study, 39 males aged 18-35 years completed an eight-week running program while consuming 60 grams per day of either colostrum or whey protein. All subjects followed dietary guidelines provided by the researchers and kept food diaries throughout the study period for subsequent dietary analysis.

Although no differences in plasma IGF-I concentrations were found between the groups at the start or end of the study, the colostrum group continued to improve its performance capacity after four weeks, while the performance of the placebo group reached a plateau. By the eighth week, the colostrum group was running further and doing more work than the placebo group. Also of note was that athletes receiving colostrum displayed a strong trend towards reducing the increase in serum creatine kinase concentrations per unit of work done, while there was no such trend in the whey group. (Creatine kinase is an enzyme that, during muscular activity, causes the breakdown of phosphocreatine in muscle to produce adenosine triphosphate (ATP), the body's energy molecule. Total creatine kinase measurement has remained the best overall marker for detection and monitoring of skeletal and muscle stress.) Injury or diseases to striated muscle most commonly cause increases in total serum creatine kinase. In this case, colostrum reduced creatine kinase levels.

Study #3: Improved Sports Performance Among Power Athletes. In another double-blind, placebo controlled trial from the

University of South Australia, 51 male power sport participants completed an eight-week standardized training program while consuming 60 grams daily of either colostrum or whey protein. The athletes were tested for power performance in a battery of tests before beginning supplementation at weeks four and eight. They followed dietary guidelines and kept food diaries throughout the trial. No additional supplementation was allowed.

The colostrum group significantly improved their maximal vertical jump heights as compared to the whey protein group. The colostrum group also improved their post-recovery vertical jump performance significantly more than the control group. Finally, the colostrum group showed greater improvements than the control group in absolute and relative peak power outputs in cycling and peak force generated by knee flexion exercises.

Study #4: Improved Performance Among Female Elite Athletes. In a double-blind, placebo controlled study, the effect of colostrum on rowing performance was studied in a group of elite female rowers. Eight female rowers from the South Australian Sports Institute completed a nine-week training program while consuming either 60 grams per day of bovine colostrum powder or whey protein powder. All subjects consumed their normal diets and kept food diaries throughout the study period.

There were significantly greater increases in the distance covered and work done by the colostrum group by week nine. Buffer capacity was also higher in the colostrum group. These results indicate that oral supplementation with bovine colostrum improves rowing performance in elite female rowers.

Colostrum for Everyone

Even if you're not the athletic type, you can still take advantage of the muscle building and metabolic benefits that are found in colostrum. The same factors which are so sought-after by athletes can contribute to weight loss and the building of lean muscle. They produce a toning and tightening effect throughout the entire body, and they can make a big difference when it comes to the ability to repair and regenerate new tissue. Studies have shown that levels of IGF-I decrease with age, but by supplementing with colostrum, the ravages of age and exercise are much less severe.

With consistent use, the growth factors in colostrum continually regenerate and rebuild the entire body. Colostrum is nature's super food—and could well prove to be as indispensable to optimal health as our daily multiple vitamin and mineral supplement.

Chapter 9

Colostrum: Protection Against NSAIDs

Aspirin, ibuprofen, diclofenac, piroxicam, naproxen. Painkillers such as these are the most commonly used drugs worldwide for treating pain and inflammation and are known as non-steroidal anti-inflammatory drugs (NSAIDs). The use of NSAIDs is routine therapy for arthritis and many other musculoskeletal disorders, as well as inflammatory conditions such as sinusitis, prostatitis, and cystitis.

Most NSAIDs can be safely used for two to three days; most are sold as over-the-counter drugs. Obviously, there are times when the use of these drugs is the best course of action. No one is calling into question their value in appropriate situations. However, using these drugs instead of, and without trying, our alternatives is a lack of healing insight. These drugs are anti-inflammatories, and they do not stimulate healing.

When these drugs are used for longer periods, virtually all patients suffer complications ranging from microbleeding and ulcers in the gastrointestinal tract to liver or kidney toxicity.

In a sense, "the cat has been let out of the bag." More than 20,000 Americans per year die from complications resulting from NSAID therapy. This is particularly true for the elderly, and for anyone with a history of peptic ulcers. In any given year, it's estimated that six percent of patients taking NSAIDs will become seriously ill and require hospitalization.

This fact was underscored in December 1998 when the Food and Drug Administration (FDA) approved the new arthritis painkiller, Celebrex. Celebrex was the first in a long-awaited new type of painkiller for millions of arthritis sufferers. It was said to be safe for the stomach, and initial sales reports show it surpassed Viagra in sales during its first month. Yet amidst all of the hype, the FDA cautioned that its stomach-safe benefits may have been overplayed.

Celebrex now bears the same warning about side-effects as many of today's standard painkillers.

Indeed, most recently Celebrex was linked to 10 deaths and 11 cases of gastrointestinal hemorrhage in its first three months on the market, according to a recent report from the *Associated Press*.

Half of the 10 people who died suffered from gastrointestinal bleeding or ulcers, according to reports submitted to the FDA that were obtained by *The Wall Street Journal* under the Freedom of Information Act. Two other deaths were attributed to heart attacks, one to drug interaction, one to a kidney disorder, and one with no cause of death listed.

Using Colostrum with NSAIDs

Because irritation to the stomach lining is so commonly associated with this broad family of drugs, many informed doctors now recommend that consumers also take first-milking colostrum.

Two important recent studies demonstrate how highly beneficial supplemental bovine colostrum can be for anyone using NSAIDs such as aspirin, ibuprofen, and other similar medications.

In an experimental study to examine whether colostrum could reduce gastrointestinal injury caused by the NSAID indomethacin (commonly used to relieve the pain, tenderness, inflammation, and stiffness caused by gout, arthritis, and other inflammatory conditions), researchers administered it together with colostrum.

As noted in the May 1999 issue of the journal *Gut*, pretreatment with colostrum reduced gastric injury by 30 to 60 percent.

The addition of colostrum to drinking water also prevented villi shortening in mice with small intestinal injuries. (Damage to villi, which are minute finger-shaped projections of the mucous membrane of the small intestine that serve in the absorption of nutrients, is an early sign of NSAID damage.) "Bovine colostrum could provide a novel, inexpensive approach for the prevention and treatment of the injurious effects of NSAIDs on the gut and may also be of value for the treatment of other ulcerative conditions of the bowel," researchers noted.

In a more recent study, researchers examined whether bovine colostrum could reduce the rise in gut permeability (a marker of intestinal injury) caused by NSAIDs in volunteers and patients taking NSAIDs for clinical reasons.

Seven healthy male volunteers participated in a randomized crossover trial comparing changes in gut permeability before and after five days of 50 mg of indomethacin three times daily together with colostrum or a placebo.

Indomethacin caused a three-fold increase in gut permeability in the placebo group, whereas no significant increase in permeability was seen when colostrum was co-administered. Therefore, the study provides "preliminary evidence that bovine colostrum, which is already currently available as an over-the-counter preparation, may provide a novel approach to the prevention of NSAID-induced gastrointestinal damage in humans," say the researchers.

How Colostrum Helps

Colostrum is a rich source of the many growth factors that aid in maintaining the integrity of the gastrointestinal tract. Human growth hormone (hGH) is the single most abundant hormone produced by the body, affecting almost every cell. Its levels are highest during the teenage years, falling rapidly thereafter, but it continues to be important in the renewal of skin, bones, and the internal tissues of the body.

Colostrum is an inexpensive, readily available source of growth factors. These growth factors have been shown to reduce gastrointestinal injury in experimental and clinical studies. Use of colostrum should also be considered for a number of other gastrointestinal conditions including ulcerative colitis, other inflammatory bowel diseases, and chemotherapy-induced mucositis.

Chapter 10

Colostrum and Dental Health

"Recently," says one of the editors of *The Doctors' Prescription for Healthy Living*, a consumer health publication, "I ran out of colostrum and experienced a delay in replenishing my supply. Do you know where I noticed the effect most? My teeth. The most immediate benefit of eating powdered colostrum was my dental health. I enjoy good dental health, but I noticed that without colostrum, my gums began to hurt."

This editor is not the only one who has noticed this effect. Researchers from the Institute of Dentistry and Turku Immunology Center at the University of Turku, Finland, have studied the benefits of colostrum on dental and oral health.

Take one recent study, when colostrum was used as a mouth rinse in a short-term human study. The colostrum had been immunized with the cavity-causing bacterium *Mutans streptococci*, creating a colostrum rich in *Mutans streptococci*-specific antibodies. Subsequently, the relative number of *Mutans streptococci* in the oral cavities of human test subjects "significantly decreased" with this special colostrum. This indicates that rinsing with bovine immune colostrum has "favorable effects" on human dental plaque, researchers say.

Bovine antibodies may also provide protection against dental caries, notes Professor Hannu Korhonen of the Agricultural Research Center, Jokioinen, Finland. "It has been shown that a colostrum-based immune milk concentrate has significant anti-metabolic potential against S. *mutans* and supports the natural antimicrobial systems present in the saliva," he says.

So far, only a few clinical human trials have been conducted on the use of anti-cavity colostrum antibodies, but Finnish researchers are encouraged. "The results obtained encourage continuation of such studies and development of innovative commercial products which contain active antibodies," says Korhonen.

Powdered Colostrum for Healthy Gums

For dental health, powdered colostrum is preferred. The tendency of first-milking colostrum to stick to the gums like a paste and dissolve is beneficial. Colostrum's growth factors and immune components work together to benefit oral health.

The same rejuvenating effects that colostrum has on the gastrointestinal membrane (see Chapter Nine) applies to the gums. The many growth factors in colostrum strengthen the lining of the gums, rejuvenating their vitality.

Wide-ranging Benefits

The human mouth is one of the main routes of entry of foreign microorganisms into the body. This is why orally transmitted diseases are widespread and common in human populations. Colostrum appears to also enhance saliva-mediated protection against dental diseases, as well as other orally transmitted infections. This has a far-reaching benefit to our health.

For example, heart disease is now known to be related to oral health. The bacterium *Porphyomonas gingivitis*, responsible for gum disease, is now also known for its damaging effects on the linings of the arteries.

This was proven by the work of Dr. Raul Garcia of the Boston VA Outpatient Clinic. As part of the VA Normative Aging Study, some

1,100 men were studied over a 25-year period. They were healthy at the start, but the men with the worst gums had twice the heart-attack rate of their peers with healthy gums and odorless breath. Their stroke rate was three times as high. The bacterium has also been found at the "scene of the crime"—in diseased carotid arteries.

By taking care of your dental health with colostrum, you're also taking care of many other aspects of your health.

Chapter 11

Colostrum and Bioterrorism

The year 1996 marked the two hundredth anniversary of Edward Jenner's first experimental vaccination—that is, inoculation with the related cowpox virus to build immunity against the deadly scourge of smallpox. For centuries, smallpox had been the greatest killer of mankind—now it may return with a vengeance if obtained by terrorists.

Dr. Jenner knew of the belief of country people that milkmaids who caught cowpox, a mild disease of cows characterized by pustular eruptions on the udders and teats, would never catch smallpox. He reasoned that if he could inoculate a person with cowpox, he could protect them from smallpox. Finally, in 1796, Dr. Jenner vaccinated a local boy, James Phipps, with cowpox taken from a milkmaid and showed that the boy was then immune to smallpox.

Clearly, colostrum enhances immune function. This alone confers greater overall immune vitality that, with proper medical care, may help to survive a bio-terrorist act. But because cows may still harbor cowpox viruses or be exposed to anthrax bacteria in the soil, colostrum may also contain minute amounts of cowpox- and anthrax-specific antibodies. While such studies have yet to be confirmed in this regard, it is reasonable to suspect that colostrum provides the passive transfer of such immune factors that may help to confer some degree of immunity upon persons who ingest this whole food concentrate.

Researchers with the Agricultural Research Center of Finland note the immunoglobulins of bovine colostrum provide the major antimicrobial protection against microbial infections and confer a passive immunity to the newborn until its own immune system matures.

But they add that immunizing cows with these pathogens or their antigens can raise the concentration in colostrum of specific antibodies against pathogens. These preparations can be used to give effective specific protection against different enteric diseases. Already, such colostral immunoglobulin supplements designed for farm animals are commercially available in many countries. Also, some immune milk products containing specific antibodies against certain pathogens have been launched for human use. A number of clinical studies are currently in progress to evaluate the efficacy of immune milks in the prevention and treatment of various human infections, including those caused by antibiotic-resistant bacteria.

But in the meantime, we know colostrum is a rich source of lactoferrin, another key protector. Lactoferrin is a mineral-binding carrier protein that attaches to available iron. Certain aerobic (growing in the presence of oxygen) bacteria, like *E. coli*, require iron to reproduce and, therefore, lactoferrin is an effective substance, when operating in the presence of a specific antibody, to impede the growth of some microorganisms in the gut. Since some forms of bioterrorism may involve tainting our food supply, these properties attributed to lactoferrin could be important. We also know lactoferrin inhibits viral replication.

"In my work as a hematologist in the former Soviet Union, I have done some research on the topic of colostrum and anthrax," notes Leonid Ber, M.D. "I found an important point for taking colostrum in this situation. It seems that anthrax causes death when it induces septic shock primarily through the action of its lethal toxin."

Chapter 12

How to Find a Quality First-milking Colostrum

Colostrum, the golden fluid that is the first mother's milk that all newborns mammals receive, is one of the most important whole foods available to consumers today. We think of it as one of nature's true gifts to the immune system, a super food, that should be a dietary staple. Colostrum is especially important for anyone interested in fighting premature aging, supporting optimal immune health, maintaining healthy muscle mass, and minimizing the typical aches and pains associated with aging.

Also known as "mother's milk," colostrum production is limited to the first few hours to the first day or two following the birth of the newborn. For bovine colostrum, which is preferred for human use because of its high potency, the highest quality is obtained within the first six hours following birth. See the resources section for a listing of quality colostrum products.

According to knowledgeable experts like Richard Cockrum, D.V.M., president of Immuno-Dynamics, there are several different forms of colostrum products available on the market today. It should be noted that not every form will impart the full benefit of colostrum to the consumer.

The three most effective products are liquid, powder and lozenges. The key—mucosal delivery system.

The science backing the use of lozenges indicates there is a much greater absorption and response of bioactive proteins. Those that do not find receptors in the lining of the mouth and throat region are protected from stomach acid and bile salts by the enzymes and hormones secreted by the salivary and other glands in the mouth and throat region.

Fresh and properly processed first-milking bovine colostrum has a pleasant, smooth taste. When incorporated into a lozenge it should look good, smell good and taste good.

The lozenge is the most effective way to utilize the benefits of colostrum. The lozenge should dwell in the mouth from 7 to 10 minutes. Why? The mouth and its associated parts or the naso-oro-pharyngeal tissues, the mucosal delivery system, are loaded with various receptors. There are greater than 50 proteins that have been isolated from first-milking bovine colostrum and many of their true biological significances have not been recognized. They are, however, recognized in the mucosal lining of the naso-oro-pharyngeal cavity and associated parts as the tongue, gingiva or the gum lines. Each part of the naso-oro-pharyngeal area has the ability to recognize very small amounts of a stimuli, pinocytosis.

The mucosal receptor-rich area is where colostrum components are recognized. When taking capsules, all of this recognition is bypassed and is deposited into a very acid stomach without buffers, added enzymes, mucous or other protectants. The acid takes its toll and it is then passed unprotected into the duodenal area of the small intestine where the bile salts and high basic digestive enzymes are.

CAPSULES

Capsules have been promoted as the premier route for administering colostrum.

When we familiarize ourselves with the gastrointestinal tract and the oro-nasal pharyngeal epithelial lining with all of its sensors, receptors, mucous glands, salivary glands, hormones, enzymes and many unknown sensors, we will become aware of some discrepancies in the capsule promotion phenomenon.

Capsules have been recommended to be taken morning, night,

with water, without water, before meals, on an empty stomach, after a meal—there is no consistency.

Capsules bypass the natural protease inhibitors, buffers, mucous secretions, hormones, enzymes, sensors and receptors and are delivered into the stomach without protection of any kind. The gelatin capsule is then dissolved and the full effects of the stomach acid are applied to the colostrum components. The components are then exposed to the rather basic bile salts in the duodenum and throughout the entire small intestine before they reach the Gut Associated Lymphoid Tissue (GALT) near the appendix, where the primary response of the capsule-ingested colostrum comes about.

Much of the colostrum components could now be altered or denatured, and diluted or rendered less effective. To compensate, a large dose of colostrum would have to be consumed to produce the same effective results.

But, the use of capsules can allow a varied quality of colostrum to be marketed.

TABLETS

Tablets have the same properties as capsules and would have the same advantages and disadvantages.

There is much said about tablets being formed under extreme pressure resulting from excessive heat.

This is a marketing "factoid" being stated. The real facts are that the binders being used to form tablets and lozenges require very little pressure, and do not destroy the full component complement in colostrum.

LOZENGES

Lozenges, which are to be held inside the mouth for several minutes, appear to be the preferred route for taking colostrum.

Why? Because the oral cavity is the gate of entry into the body's communication network. As a child, calf, foal, puppy or kitten nurses the lacteal secretion, colostrum floods the oro-nasal pharyngeal cavity, exposing the secretion to the many receptor sites. These receptor sites form a variety of communication pathways that distribute signals to various parts of the body.

Part of the pharyngeal region contains lymphoid cells, tonsils, referred to as MALT, Mucosal Associated Lymphoid Tissue. This is the same type of tissue as the lymphoid tissue near the illio-cecal valve termed as GALT, Gut Associated Lymphoid Tissue, discussed in the capsule section.

The great advantage of MALT over GALT is that MALT is present early on, before any digestive processes start to alter the colostral components as in GALT. MALT is also protected by many of the buffers, enzymes, mucous and other protective properties secreted by glands in the oro-naso pharyngeal lamina propria.

Studies have been done on the effects of cytokine, for instance, interferon alpha IF2 in combating stress and exposure to disease when presented orally. Large doses were not as effective as smaller doses. This indicates that grossly more is not better.

The purpose of taking colostrum is to aid in normalizing and regulating normal body function, and in particular, the immune system.

Resources

Health Direct
320 Kalmus Drive
Costa Mesa, California 92626
(800) 597-0078, Dept. CGB
www.healthdirectusa.com

None of the nutritional treasures in colostrum are available at desirable peak concentrations unless consumers choose true first-milking colostrum. Colostrum Gold™ from Health Direct is one of the very best and truest first-milking colostrum products available today.

Immune-Tree
1163 S. 1680 W.
Orem, Utah 84058
(888) 484-8671
www.immunetree.com

Immune-Tree offers a full line of guaranteed first-milking colostrum products for every lifestyle, including children's chewables, pineapple lozenges, capsules, and powder.

Garden of Life
770 North Point Parkway
West Palm Beach, Florida 33407
(800) 622-8986
www.gardenoflifeusa.com

Goatein™ IG is the only goat's milk protein colostrum formula on the market today. The goats are not fed pesticides, herbicides, growth hormones or antibiotics. Goatein IG can be taken by many people who can't tolerate cow's milk products.

Receive a FREE Trial Issue of Healthy Living

Keep up with the latest findings in health and healing from top health experts and receive a free trial issue of Healthy Living, the nation's leading consumer health publication today.

Just mail, fax, e-mail, or call us with your mailing information.

SEND TO:
Healthy Living Free Trial Offer
1801 Chart Trail
Topanga, California 90290
FAX TO: (310) 455-8962
CALL TOLL-FREE: (800) 959-9797
E-MAIL TO:
info@freedompressonline.com

Visit Healthy Living at www.freedompressonline.com.

References

CHAPTER 3

Orzechowska, B., et al. "Antiviral effect of proline-rich polypeptide in murine resident peritoneal cells." Acta Virol; 1998;42(2):75-78.

Wieczorek, Z., et al. "Proline-rich polypeptide from ovine colostrum: its effect on skin permeability and on the immune response." *Immunology*, 1979;36(4):875-881.

CHAPTER 4

Any detergent ending in eth, as in sodium laureth sulfate, or "PEG" compounds, are likely to be contamianted with 1,4-dioxane.

"Are hair dyes safe?" *Consumer Reports*, August 1979: 455-460.

Examples of carcinogenic dyes: diamonotoluene, diaminoanisole, and others which are phenylenediamine-based.

Examples of artificial colors: CI Disperse Blue No. 1 and Red No. 33.

Federal Register, August 30, 1988; 53(168): 33110-33121.

Federal Register, September 28, 1982; 47(188): 42563-42566.

Food and Drug Administration (FDA). *Cosmetic Handbook*. (undated).

Habel, L.A., et al. "Occupational exposures and risk of breast cancer in middle-aged women." International Conference on Women's Health: Occupation & Cancer, November 1-2, 1993, National Institutes of Health.

Johnasen, M. & Bundgaard, H. "Kinetics of formaldehyde release from the cosmetic preservative Germall 115. Arch. Pharm. Chem. Sci., 1981; 9: 117-122.

Mickleson, KN, Moriarty, KM "Immunoglobulin levels in human colostrum and milk."J. Pediatr Gastroenterol Nutr. 1(3):381-4 1982.

National Cancer Institute (NCI). "Bioassay of 2,4-diaminotoluene for possible carcinogenicity." *Carcinogenesis Technical Report Series, no. 162, 1979*.

National Cancer Institute (NCI). "Bioassay of 2,4-diaminoanisole sulfate for possible carcinogenicity." *Carcinogenesis Technical Report Series, no. 84, 1978*.

"Nitrosamine-contaminated cosmetics; call for industry action; request for data." Federal Register, April 10, 1979; 44(70): 21365.

Office of Population Censuses and Surveys. Occupational Mortality Decennial Supplement, 1979-80, 1982-83, 1986. Great Britain, London, Her Majesty's Stationery Office, as cited in IARC Monographs Volume 57.

Pukkala, E. et al. "Changing cancer risk patterns among Finnish hairdressers." *Int. Arch. Occup. Environ. Health*, 1992; 64: 39-42.

Rojanapo, W., et al. "Carcinogenicity of an oxidation product of p-phenylenediamine." Carcinogenesis, 1986, 17(12): 1997-2002.

Rump, JA; et al. "Treatment of diarrhea in human immunodeficiency virus-infected patients with immunoglobulin from bovine colostrum." Clin Investig Jul;70(7):588-94.

Steinman, D. & Epstein, S.S. *The Safe Shopper's Bible*, New York, NY: Macmillan, 1995.

Steinman, D. Regarding carcinogenicity testing on 4-EMPD. FOI Request No. F94-7549, March 16, 1994. Food and Drug Administration, Washington, D.C.

The commonest carcinogenic metals are cobalt, lead, and nickel.

The commonest carcinogenic petrochemicals are dyes such as Red No. 9, Acid Orange 87, and Solvent Brown 44.

The commonest nitrosamine-forming detergents are diethanolamine and triethanolamine.

The commonest formaldehy-releasing preservatives are imidazolidinyl urea, diazolidinyl urea, quaternium 15, 2-bromo-2-nitropropane-1,3-diol, and DMDM hydantoin.

Winter, R. *A Consumer's Dictionary of Cosmetic Ingredients*, New York, NY: Crown Publishers, 1989, p. 120.

Winter, R. *A Consumer's Dictionary of Cosmetic Ingredients*, New York, NY: Crown Publishers, 1989, p. 256.

CHAPTER 5

Cummings, NP; et al. "Oxidative metabolic response and microbial activity of human milk macrophages: Effect of lipopolysaccharide and muramyl dipeptide." Infect Immun Aug;49(2):435-9. 1985.

Huppertz, HI; et al. "Bovine colostrum ameliorates diarrhea in infection with diarrheagenic Escherichia coli, shiga toxin-producing E. coli, and E coli expressing intimin and hemolysin." J Pediatr Gastroenterol Nutr. Oct;29(4):452-6. 1999.

Lissner, R.; et al. "A standard immunoglobulin preparation produced from bovine colostra shows antibody reactivity and neutralization activity against Shiga-like toxins and EHEC-hemolysin of Escherichia coli O157:H7." Infection Sep-Oct;24(5):378-83. 1996.

Plettenberg, A; et al. "A preparation from bovine colostrum in the treatment of HIV-positive patients with chronic diarrhea." Clin Investig Jan;71(1):42-5. 1993.

Stephan, W; et al. "Antibodies from colostrum in oral immunotherapy." Clin Chem Clin Biochem Jan;28(1): 19-23. 1990.

CHAPTER 6

Ebina, T., et al. "Treatment of multiple sclerosis with anti-measles cow colostrum." Med Microbiol Immunol (Berl), 1984;173(2):87-93.

Ferrante, P., et al. "[Serum and cerebrospinal fluid antibodies against measles virus in patients with multiple sclerosis.]" Arch Sci Med (Torino), 1982;139(1):39-43.

Meilants, H. "Reflections on the link between intestinal permeability and inflammatory joint disease." Clin Exp Rheumatology, 1990;8(5):523-524.

Ohara, Y. "Multiple sclerosis and measles virus." Jpn J Infect Dis, 1999;52(5):198-200.

The Burton Goldberg Group. *Alternative Medicine: The Definitive Guide.* Puyallup, WA: Future Medicine Publishing, Inc., p. 531.

Webster, H.D. "Growth factors and myelin regeneration in multiple sclerosis." Mult Scler, 1997;3(2):113-120.

CHAPTER 7

Carroll PV et al. "rhIgF-1 administration reduces insulin requirements, decreases growth hormone secretion, and improves the lipid profile in adults with IDDM." Diabetes 1997 Sep;46(9):1453-8

Cowley, G. "A New Way to Fight Diabetes," *Newsweek* Nov. 15, 1993.

Dohm, G. L., et al. "IgF-1 stimulated glucose transport in human skeletal muscle and IgF-1 resistance in obesity and NIDDM." Diabetes, 1990;39(9):1028-1032.

Nam Sy, et al. "Low-dose growth hormone treatment combined with diet restriction decreases insulin resistance by reducing visceral fat and increasing muscle mass in obese type 2 diabetic patients." Int J Obes Relat Metab Disord, 2001;25(8):1101-1107.

Pennisi. "Immune therapy stems diabetes progress," *Science News*, January 15,1995;45:37.

Staroscik, K., et al. "Immunologically active nonapeptide fragment of a proline-rich polypeptide from bovine colostrum: amino acid sequence and immuno-regulatory properties." Molecular Immunology, 1983; 20(12):1277-1282.

CHAPTER 8

Buckley, J., et al. "Effect of an oral bovine colostrum supplement (intact TM) on running performance." Abstract from: 1998 Australian Conference of Science and Medicine in Sport, Adelaide, South Australia, October 1998.

Buckley, J., et al. ""Oral supplementation with bovine colostrum (intact TM) increases vertical jump performance." Presented at 4th Annual Congress of the European College of Sports Science, Rome 14-17 July, 1999.

Mero, A., et al. "Effects of bovine colostrum supplementation on serum IGF-I, IgG, hormone, and saliva IgA during training." J Appl Physiol, 1997;83(4):144-1151.

Wu, A.H. & Perryman, M.B. "Clinical applications of muscle enzymes and proteins." Curr Opin Rheumatol, 1992;4(6):815-820.

CHAPTER 9

Fries, J., et al. "Adverse drug reactions, surveillance." Arthritis, Rheumatology, 1991; 34: 1353-1360.

"FDA approves new pain-killer for arthritis." Associated Press, December 31, 1998.

Lazarou, P., et al. "Incidence of adverse drug reactions in hospitalized patients; meta-analysis of prospective studies." Journal of the American Medical Association, 1998; 279: 1200-1204.

Playford, R.J., et al. "Bovine colostrum is a health food supplement which prevents NSAID induced gut damage." Gut,1999;44(5):653-658.

Playford, R.J., et al. "Co-administration of the health food supplement, bovine colostrum, reduces the acute non-steroidal anti-inflammatory drug-induced increase in intestinal permeability." Clin Sci (Lond), 2001;100(6):627-633.

The Associated Press. "Report: Celebrex linked to 10 deaths." April 20, 1999.

CHAPTER 10

Loimaranta, V., et al. "Effects of bovine immune and non-immune whey preparations on the com position and pH response of human dental plaque." Eur J Oral Sci, 1999;107(4):244-250.

CHAPTER 11

"Antiviral effect of bovine lactoferrin saturated with metal ions on early steps of human immunod eficiency virus type 1 infection." Int J Biochem Cell Biol, 1998;30(9):1055-1062.

"Cowpox," Microsoft® Encarta® Online Encyclopedia 2000 http://encarta.msn.com © 1997-2000 Microsoft Corporation.

Hagiwara, K., et al. "Detection of cytokines in bovine colostrum." Vet Immunol Immunopathol, 2000;76(3-4):183-190.

Hanna, P.C., et al. "On the role of macrophages in anthrax." Proc Natl Acad Sci U S A, 1993;90(21):10198-10201.

Korhonen, H., et al. "Bovine milk antibodies for health." Br J Nutr, 2000;84(Suppl 1): S135-S146.

Index

The Colostrum Miracle